Nancy J. Bladen

LIVING WELL

LIVING

A
Twelve-Step
Response
to
Chronic
Illness
and
Disability

by
Martha Cleveland

WELL

1817

A HARPER/HAZELDEN BOOK

HARPER & ROW, PUBLISHERS, SAN FRANCISCO

New York, Cambridge, Philadelphia, St. Louis
London, Singapore, Sydney, Tokyo

FIRST HARPER & ROW EDITION PUBLISHED IN 1989.

Library of Congress Cataloging-in-Publication Data

Cleveland, Martha.
　Living well.

　"A Harper/Hazelden book"
　Bibliography: p.
　Includes index.
　1. Chronic diseases—Psychological aspects.　I. Title.
RC108.C54　1989　　　155.9′16　　　88-45995
ISBN 0-06-255416-6

89　90　91　92　93　MCN　10　9　8　7　6　5　4　3　2　1

To my husband, Walter, and my children, Mark, Jayne, and David—who have unfailingly and lovingly supported me, all of our time together.

ACKNOWLEDGMENTS

I find there is really no way to sort out the impact and influence that my life experiences, loved ones, friends, colleagues, and associates have had on this book. But I want to acknowledge a few people who directly stand out. My husband and children, who are the bedrock. Dr. Paul Rosenblatt, teacher, advisor, and mentor, who assumed that I could think, write, and publish what I had written. Christina Baldwin, whose professional encouragement taught me to put aside the protection of clinical jargon and write as myself. Dr. John Bergman, dermatologist, friend, and human being, whose expertise, attention, care, and respect have made my life with alopecia much less lonely. All of my friends and colleagues who have supported me in this work, particularly the staff of the Family Therapy Institute in St. Paul. And finally the editorial staff at Hazelden Educational Materials—Judy Delaney, Jeff Petersen, and all the hidden others whose perceptive comments and questions have shaped and deepened this work. To all of you, many, many thanks.

The vignettes in this book are composites based on the experiences of chronically ill and disabled people. Any resemblance to actual persons, living or dead, or specific situations, is entirely coincidental.

—The Editors

CONTENTS

Introduction	Joy Will Come in the Morning	1
Chapter One	"Our Wound Is the Place . . ."	5
Chapter Two	Who's Challenged?	11
Chapter Three	What's the Problem?	15
Chapter Four	The Twelve Step Journey	31
Chapter Five	Gaining Strength Through New Beliefs	47
Chapter Six	Taking an Inventory	57
Chapter Seven	Pain to be Found and Faced	61
Chapter Eight	Consequences of Unfaced Pain	83
Chapter Nine	Filling the Void with Positives	87
Chapter Ten	Taking Our Struggle to the Outside World	95
Chapter Eleven	Making Amends	111
Chapter Twelve	Spiritual Awakening	121
Chapter Thirteen	Gaining Peace	127
Chapter Fourteen	What Will Happen	137

Appendix One   The Twelve Steps for
                   Chronically Ill or Disabled People 145

Appendix Two   The Twelve Steps of
                   Alcoholics Anonymous 146

Appendix Three Daily Meditations 147

Appendix Four Finding a Mutual Aid Group 149

Bibliography 152

Index 153

LIVING WELL

JOY WILL COME
IN THE MORNING

I was 33 years old when I first got really sick. I felt exhausted, depressed, with aching joints and fingernails that kept splitting and peeling off. My blood counts showed that something was wrong, but none of the doctors could say exactly what it was. Then I lost my hair. All of it. Every hair on my body fell out. They called it Alopecia Universalis. I was grotesque, a freak. One doctor, a psychiatrist, wanted to take my picture for a textbook and I was so ashamed, anxious, and insecure that I almost let him. I shudder to think how I would have felt, knowing that for generations to come medical students would see me as some kind of human aberration.

I was told that the medical profession had no remedy, that all of this was probably due to emotional stress, that it was up to me to relax. I cried a lot, raged some, felt helpless, hopeless, alone, and terrified. My days buzzed with anxiety; my nights were filled with dreams of screaming and suffocating. But my husband and children needed me and my friends kept calling, so I put on an awful wig and crept back into life. Two years later my hair came back, but my blood counts remained abnormal and things were never to be the same.

As I grew older my hair fell out again, and then again, and still no help was available. Not only was there no medical aid, but there was no emotional support from my doctors either. They didn't know how to fix my body and weren't trained to deal with my soul.

When I was fifty, I finally went to a well-known rheumatologist (a specialist in muscle and joint diseases) who said, "It's not stress, not basically anyway; your body doesn't work right. You've got a physical problem. I can tell you what's wrong, but I can't do anything for you. There's something haywire with your immune system, and we don't know much about immune systems. Some day we'll be able to treat people like you with something, much like we treat diabetics today, but for now all I can do is say that something *is* wrong and it's not your fault."

That was eight years ago. Again I cried, but this time with relief and gratitude. Then I began the long road to understanding how to live with a chronic illness.

Of health care problems in the United States today, some 80 percent relate to chronic illness or disability, Daniel Anderson, Ph.D., tells us in *Living with a Chronic Illness*. There are a lot of us out here, and while the medical community helps manage our acute episodes, it is not structured to give us the kind of support we need over the months and years we live with our condition. And live with it we must. Whether it's a physical problem that life has dealt us, such as chronic heart disease, a nervous system disorder, cancer, diabetes, autoimmune disease, or perhaps a major emotional impairment such as schizophrenia or manic-depressive psychosis, we sometimes feel that our situation is unbearable.

Dr. Anderson tells us that how we bear our unbearable is largely our choice, and that too often our response creates as much stress as the disease or disability itself. In our confusion, fear, and anger, we may react in ways that limit us and leave us living diminished lives. But we can change this. While we can't alter the fact that our chronic illness and disability may never be healed, we can learn to live in a way that reduces stress on ourselves and those around us, stops making our physical problems worse, and helps us to become happier, more productive people.

I believe that most people with chronic illness or disability suffer also from intense and chronic emotional pain. This pain equals and often surpasses the physical pain or disablement caused by our condition. We may feel lonely, angry, depressed, or hopeless, and feelings of isolation and powerlessness begin to set the boundaries of our lives. In our emotional pain we may reduce our involvement with family, friends, and work. Then people tell us that our emotional struggles can make our chronic condition worse, so we add to our load by blaming ourselves for not relaxing and accepting things as they are. In our heart of hearts, we know that we have only this one life to live, and we yearn to become the very most we can be in the time we have. And sometimes it is terribly hard to remember that, whatever our physical or mental limitations, we are incomparable individuals who can make a unique contribution to our world. While we can't control the reality of our illness or disability, we *can* choose how to respond emotionally and spiritually to that reality.

The Alcoholics Anonymous recovery program offers a unique method to recover from our emotional pain, a method we will explore in this book. A.A. is a program originally developed by alcoholics for alcoholics to help themselves and each other recover from their self-destructive behavior. It is now a worldwide organization that touches millions of lives. The core of A.A. is the Twelve Steps, which can be "worked" one day at a time. As recovering alcoholics work the program, as they study, interpret, and integrate its beliefs and behaviors into their lives, they are "in recovery." This recovery process is a lifetime commitment.

The Twelve Step program is spiritual, based on action coming from love, and has been the only truly effective method of dealing with alcoholism. In addition to being used in the treatment of alcoholics, it is now applied in treating other addictions such as eating, gambling, and drugs other than alcohol. I believe it can also treat the emotional pain connected with chronic illness and disability.

A.A. is directed toward spiritual growth. By adapting this program to our unique situations and applying its principles to our individual lives, we can outmaneuver the effects of our physical illness with spiritual wellness. This is not an easy process; it won't work without serious commitment and a willingness to change our behaviors as well as our belief systems. But if we truly trust in the recovery process, things *do* change. Our feelings of depression and isolation can lift as we find a spiritual common ground with others who share our experience. Our hatred of powerlessness can change as we learn to accept the unmanageability of our bodies. This way, we can transform powerlessness into a tool that can help us find peace in our lives. No matter what our physical or mental limitations, we can work toward a fulfilled life, one lived without fear, shame, or loneliness and supported by love, serenity, and joy.

It is the premise of this book that we do not have ultimate control over our bodies, and that we may spend our lives living with a chronic illness or disability. But we do have control over the fulfillment of our spiritual potential.

I hope that this small book can help others who live with chronic illness or disability. In the first three chapters I have explained the problem as I have come to see it through my own experience and work with others. Chapters Four through Thirteen take you through the Twelve Steps of A.A., redefined here so each Step becomes especially meaningful to us. Chapter Fourteen is a hopeful prophecy, describing what the outcome of our commitment to spiritual wellness can be. Finally, I have included a list of the Twelve Steps, a daily meditation, and information about contacting a mutual aid group.

An old Negro spiritual tells us, "Weeping may endure for a night, but joy will come in the morning." Let that morning be ours.

CHAPTER ONE

"OUR WOUND IS THE PLACE . . ."

Our wound is the place where our soul finds entry into us. The calamity that strikes may be our call to spiritual fulfillment.

— *Ernest Lawrence Rossi*

In the beginning there were two perfect people—a perfect man named Adam and a perfect woman named Eve. They lived in a garden full of light and trees and flowers, and they glowed with health and beauty. The serpent, whose name was Reality, lay coiled behind a rock, unseen and unheeded. After a while Reality got tired of being ignored and slid through time and the woods into another garden.

Here things were different. The sun shined, trees grew, and flowers bloomed, but clouds dotted the blue sky and a few weeds sprouted among the blossoms. The people were different too. Some were bent, some blind, some sat in wheelchairs, and some stood tall with faces that showed pain and suffering. This garden was Reality's home.

Perhaps it's from these conflicting images that we look at our world. We know where Reality lives, but we may act as if Reality doesn't exist. We may honor beauty and reject imperfection. We have beauty pageants and may pretend that a contestant's talents matter in the judging. But most of us believe that what wins is the perfect face, the shiny hair, the slender legs, and the sexy body in a bathing suit. Our television personalities and politicians—people who help shape the way we view our world—may be painted, coiffed, sprayed, and color coded to one-dimensional perfection. It's easy for us to blame advertising and the media, but they only offer us what we may want so badly: physical and mental perfection. We may tell ourselves that if we look well-groomed and healthy, if we don't show or talk about afflictions, then we are good, worthwhile people who belong. The tragedy is that this leaves a society of mostly imperfect people trying to become perfect—and pushing those who are obviously unable to meet the criteria outside of the boundaries.

And what about those of us who are not perfect, who don't glow with health and beauty, who are in some way different? As children we may have learned that to have a physical imperfection is not "normal." To be injured is acceptable only if we cry about it as little as possible, if it heals quickly, and if it doesn't leave scar tissue. A child unlucky enough to be born with a physical or mental differentness is taught while still very young to hide or disguise his difference—and as he learns this, he also learns to be ashamed of himself.

Those of us who develop chronic illness or disabilities later in life have also learned these lessons. All our lives we may have been taught not to stare, or that we should ignore another's difference. So when we become afflicted, we feel as though we are joining a group of people who are somehow undesirable and outside the normal boundaries of society. We become defined by our wound, our illness or disability, and many of us come to believe that definition. We use up our emotional energies in our struggle to prove ourselves to others, to pass, or pretend, or in some other way to be just like everyone else. In this struggle to hide or reject our differentness, we forget that it is part of us and that if we reject it, we end up rejecting our total self.

From Darkness to Light

Our culture loses much by refusing to honor the darker things in life. Wounds and shadows can offer great gifts. For one thing, they offer balance. They allow us to see life whole. When we think about it, most of life's meaning is defined in terms of contrasts. We can't really experience light unless we have known darkness; we don't know what sweet is until we taste sour. When we fill a white bowl with red petunias, the red becomes more brilliant, the white clearer. Joy often rises from sadness, and love is more precious when we know what it is to hate.

Wise people throughout the ages have written that we can't truly and fully live life until we have accepted our own mortality. How often, when our lives or the lives of our loved ones are threatened, we yearn for the treasure of a quiet walk, a few minutes in a favorite chair with the cat curled in our lap, an uneventful evening of TV, or a hot bath and a good book. Time and time again we hear from terminally ill people that in knowing they are going to lose life, they find its meaning and cherish each moment of the time that they have. The same insight comes to many of us who become chronically ill or disabled. Somehow the loss of complete health or full physical function shakes us up and our priorities settle in a different order. As we question our future, we learn to live more completely in the present; we give and take from life without assuming there will be a tomorrow and another tomorrow; and we stop taking life for granted and start noticing it.

Also, accepting and understanding wounds and shadows releases us from fear. When we are able to live openly with the imperfections of ourselves and others, they become familiar companions rather than frightening specters to be hidden or denied. How much easier to say, "I have cancer," or "I shake because I have Parkinson's disease," than to make up excuses about baldness or fatigue or a trembling hand. How much more comfortable it is to be able to say, "Can I help you?" to the woman in a wheelchair struggling to open a restaurant door, than to hold back, not knowing what to do, afraid to hurt her feelings. When we deny our illnesses or disabilities by pretending they don't exist, we make them shameful, and we give them the power to make us afraid. Only recognizing and accepting them can free us from our fear.

Finally, physical and emotional wounds offer a place for our souls to enter. This doesn't mean that people without illnesses or disabilities are without souls; the point is that without facing the realities of impairment, it's easier to deny spiritual development and spend our energy chasing physical perfection. Yet how often we hear someone who has faced, or is living in, a serious crisis say, "It's awful, but I've learned about what's important in life and have seen how to make life better for me."

Psychology tells us that it's change in life's circumstances that brings about changes in people. When lives are disrupted, people have to move, to be somehow different in order to adapt to the new situation. When we are disabled or chronically ill, we are faced with a challenge: How are we going to handle this? What direction will our change take?

Our Spirits Are Still Ours

For those of us who live with chronic illness or disability the challenge is clear. Our bodies are no longer predictable, our trust in our physical self is shaken, and nature seems out of control. But our spirits are still ours and will always be ours. Spiritual fulfillment can be our goal, and our souls can support and guide us on whatever path our bodies take.

It's very hard to define individual human spirituality. Just as we think we have come up with an explanation, some part of it eludes us. Some people believe in an external, personal God, a force outside of themselves. For them, spiritual growth and fulfillment come through a strengthening relationship with this God. Others recognize an impersonal Power or Force greater than themselves where they can turn for help as they struggle with their lives. Still others find spiritual development in their individual integrity and their interaction with the universe.

Whatever approach they take, people reach spiritual fulfillment by attending to, and expanding, the life force within them. Our spirituality is our essence, our energy toward living. To grow spiritually is to use that energy in a positive way, so that both our own lives and the lives of those around us are enriched. Spiritual wellness can mean becoming the very best human being we can be. M. Scott Peck, in *The Road Less Traveled,* tells us that love is the will to extend ourselves for the purpose of nurturing our own or someone else's spiritual growth. So when we commit ourselves to spiritual growth we commit ourselves to love. This is a lifelong process; there is never a point where we graduate to some higher state of permanent fulfillment. But if we dedicate ourselves to spiritual growth, and if we truly believe in the potential of our spirit, we will come to be full of life and at peace with that fullness.

When we are disabled or chronically ill, our spirit is tested. It can be crushed, leading to rage, desperation, or despair. Or it can be challenged, leading us to love, acceptance, and serenity. The choice is ours. Even if our physical condition seems out of control, we can choose how to react to our illness or disability. We can see it as a threat or as a challenge. We can become shriveled, mean, with eyes always looking inward. Or we can stretch, reach out, becoming all that we can be with everything we have. Frances H. Burnett, in *The Secret Garden,* a beautiful book about overcoming illness and grief, has the old gardener tell the children that thistles can't grow where roses are cultivated—and this is true. We can let our thistles grow, or we can choose to nurture roses.

CHAPTER TWO

WHO'S CHALLENGED?

If this were the best of all possible worlds, society would be challenged to change its beliefs about imperfection and differentness. Unfortunately, even if this should happen, it would be a long, slow process, and there is an urgent, present need to deal with the day-to-day reality of the chronically ill and disabled. So who's challenged?

The answer is—anyone. Anyone can be challenged by a disease, a freak accident, a birth defect, the wrong combination of genes, or the physical or mental breakdowns that come with aging. Our group contains people of both sexes, people of all ages from infancy through the very old, Black, Caucasian, Asian, Christians, Jews, Mohammedans, and atheists. Who you are or where you come from simply doesn't matter—if the challenge comes, it comes, regardless.

Some of us are challenged by a disability that shows: it is clear for the world to see.

Senator Daniel Inouye of Hawaii makes no attempt to hide his missing arm. My blind mother feels her way across the room with her cane extended to warn her of obstacles. A young male paraplegic maneuvers his wheelchair through a crowded aisle in the discount store. An acquaintance fiddles with her hearing aid. The child in front of you turns her head and you may be shocked by the Down's syndrome showing on her face.

Many others walk with hidden illnesses.

The woman next to you in the grocery checkout line has cancer in her stomach. There is no way you can know. Your business associate quietly takes his blood pressure medication at lunch and studies the menu for low-salt, low-fat food. He doesn't comment, and no one notices. A recovering alcoholic lawyer nurses a soft drink at the cocktail party. The older woman next to you in the theater shifts in her seat as she tries to still the raging pain in her hip. Her quick frown seems meaningless.

And in addition to those who carry hidden illness or disability, there are all the others who love and care for them.

The woman in the grocery checkout line has a cancer that is not only hers but her family's. Her husband wonders about how he can support her and take care of their home while she is ill from chemotherapy. Her children watch her, afraid she will die and leave them. All of them think about how her illness means putting aside their own needs in life. The young paraplegic's mother worries that he won't marry and know the joy of fathering a child. His father is afraid that his son will never feel like a man. His girlfriend is caught between her love for him and her grief in giving up her dream of a perfect husband. The recovering alcoholic lawyer's wife secretly watches him at the party, pushing aside her fear that he might drink again.

These people are challenged too.

When people are struck with chronic illnesses or disabilities, they tend to feel powerless. But for family and friends the situation is very different. From the moment of onset, the person with the illness or disability gains great power. Family life becomes organized around the needs and limitations of the chronically ill or disabled person. When a paraplegic adolescent comes home from the rehab hospital the structure of the house has to be changed. Ramps are built, doors widened, and bedrooms re-arranged so that his care is more convenient for the caregivers. Special foods may be necessary; a routine for all of the demanding physical care must be worked out. His paraplegia becomes the situation around which the entire family is organized. His physical condition and emotional state are the central focus of the family. The disabled person has never had so much power.

The same sort of changes occur with friends too. Friends of the parents rally around to help, but it's hard to talk about things other than the son's disability and all that it involves. It is an unnatural situation, one for which there aren't clear rules for behavior. The same is true for the adolescent's friends. Some remain in contact, but many stay away because they don't know what to say or do, and are afraid of saying or doing the wrong thing. Siblings' relationships are disrupted too. There are a lot fewer after-school or overnight visits at their house than there were when the paraplegic was just a big brother.

Common Realities

The form and prognosis of disability and chronic illness differ greatly. Some disabilities such as blindness, deafness, and para-plegia are physically limiting but not life-threatening, and life-styles can be moderated to accommodate them. Some conditions, such as diabetes and most hypertension, are controllable with medication, diet, and stress reduction. Some illnesses that have been chronic for years can be cured by the discovery of a new drug, or even occasionally by a religious or spiritual experience. But most illnesses cannot, and must be managed through periods of remission and during times when the disease is active.

Despite differences in the forms and eventual outcomes of chronic illness and disability, they all result in some common realities for those who have them. All of us lose some kind of function; all of us are in some way restricted. Freedom of choice and flexibility are reduced in our lives. To a greater or lesser degree the illness or disability controls us and sets the boundaries for our thoughts, feelings, and actions. And we all suffer emotional pain.

This is where the challenge comes in. First, we are challenged to create our individual response to the uncertainty and limitations of our social and emotional lives. Second, and perhaps even more difficult, is the struggle to sustain our self-esteem in a society that sees us as different and somehow second class. Third, we may feel pressure to make others comfortable with our limitations. In social relationships between disabled and nondisabled people, the disabled often must carry the burden of managing the situation so that the "normal" people are not anxious or upset.

As we are challenged, each of us is forced to change. We may stretch or we may shrink, but we can't not change. We can choose to increasingly allow our lives to revolve around our physical condition. Or we can choose to commit ourselves to spiritual growth, refusing to let our physical condition limit the boundaries of our soul. We can choose to have spiritual health overcome physical illness or disablement.

The second choice sounds great, but how do we do it? Commitment to spiritual growth is not easy. Old habits, old ways of feeling and responding trip us up over and over. And there is no final fulfillment, no ultimate goal that is ever attained. But in our struggle toward spiritual wellness we find little miracle after little miracle, and one day serenity may surprise us. We may think, *Things are different. I am different. I am happy. I feel peace.* The feeling may not stay with us for long, but once we have had it, our reality has shifted in a deep and basic way and we have permanently changed. Our choice has taken hold.

For chronically ill and disabled people who choose this way, the question is, "What are the obstacles we face if we choose our souls over our bodies? We clearly understand what our bodies struggle against, but what stands in the way of our spirit?"

CHAPTER THREE

WHAT'S THE PROBLEM?

When you live with a chronic illness or a disability, "What's the problem?" looks like a pretty silly question. There are so many. Physically, our lives are limited to one degree or another; we tend to think a lot about our condition and often need to plan our lives around it. In many cases this is realistic. There *are* things we can or cannot do or eat or expect.

Yet many of us believe that our limits are the central focus of how we live, and we allow realistic limitations to spread unrealistically into areas of our lives where they don't belong.

A man with chronic heart problems may become so focused on his situation that he limits his exercise and relationships so that he won't unnecessarily stress himself. Or perhaps he goes to the other extreme, spending hours walking, running, and playing tennis while avoiding a social life so that he won't be faced with tempting food and drink. An older woman who loses her sight can no longer tell where the food is on her plate. But this real limitation is extended to become I can't go to a restaurant because I can't see my food. *This then extends to* My life is so restricted, what's the use of it all? *A woman having chemotherapy loses her hair, hates how she looks in a wig, and stops socializing with her friends. A middle-aged male diabetic is impotent and avoids physical intimacy with his wife.*

All kinds of conditions, all kinds of solutions—but all are solutions primarily related to the physical part of us. Or are they?

In this chapter we will discuss the problems chronically ill and disabled people face. We will attempt to identify the sources of their emotional pain. Then in Chapter Four we will show how to cope with that emotional pain and how it can be alleviated.

Basically, the way we behave in response to our illnesses or disabilities is based on pain—but the pain may be emotional, not physical. We who are in some way or another impaired share chronic, sometimes overwhelming, emotional pain. We fear our condition will get worse; many of us fear that it will kill us. At times we feel helpless, hopeless, trapped, even desperate. We may become depressed, grieving for the selves that we aren't; we may become rageful, thinking, *I hate it, I hate it, make it go away.* We may be ashamed and isolate ourselves, believing that we are worthless and that no one can understand. We can become exhausted from trying to cope. The intensity of emotional pain varies from person to person, and some of us are more troubled by one kind than another, but we *all* experience it.

That emotional pain can contribute to our spiritual development seems contradictory. By itself, it would seem to destroy spirituality. In her lovely pamphlet, *Shame Faced*, Stephanie E. says that spirituality and shame cannot coexist, that negative emotions can diminish or destroy our spirits. Yet others tell us that in confronting and struggling with emotional pain our spirits are strengthened and expanded. So our emotional pain is both our curse and our blessing. But it's hard to look at it this way; it may *feel* like a curse.

Identifying Our Emotional Pain

One of our first tasks in dealing with emotional pain is to identify it and place it in context. We'll now discuss common emotional pains chronically ill and disabled people face, and show briefly how each can be turned into a positive experience.

Powerlessness

Both chronic illnesses and disabilities can be uncontrollable, and chronic illness is often unpredictable as well. A deaf man cannot hear, a young woman with systemic lupus erythematosus (a disorder of the immune system) does not know what the course of her disease will be. So when we become ill or disabled, our feelings of loss of control are based on reality. But early in our life we have learned that to be in control means to be safe: our very survival depends on it.

And now, perhaps suddenly, we can no longer control the most basic thing in our life—our body. Loss of control feels like powerlessness, and our feelings of powerlessness may lead to feelings of helplessness, hopelessness, rage, and even panic or despair. Also, our self-esteem seems to decrease in direct proportion to the increase in our sense of powerlessness. It is not unusual for a disabled or chronically ill person to feel hopeless about life and think, *What good is life if I can't be like other people?* or to despair, *How can I feel like life is worth anything at all when I have to depend so much on other people?* And many of us may become anxious or panic-stricken. We may be miserably uncomfortable but still hide the more devastating feeling of being worthless or having no control in our lives.

As we feel less and less powerful we become more and more preoccupied with maintaining control over both our internal life and our external world. We may try to manipulate and control everything and as a consequence revert to a preoccupation with ourselves. We may use any tool possible to gain a feeling of control, even sometimes playing on others' guilt in order to manipulate them. We may hate ourselves for doing this, but it *is* a kind of power. Frequently, we don't give ourselves credit for the healthy gains in control that we do make.

A stroke patient learns to take five steps without help—for a few moments she feels triumphant, then quickly says, "That's

*not so much. What does it really matter? I'll probably never
be able to go up and down the stairs at home."*

Powerlessness may seem like a total curse—what blessing
could it possibly bestow? In Chapter Four, when we begin to
examine the Twelve Steps and how chronically ill and disabled
people can use them to enrich their lives, we will find that
acceptance of powerlessness is a basic first step on the journey
toward spiritual wellness. What seems to be our most basic
emotional pain—the pain on which all our other pain is built
— can become our ticket to freedom.

Fear and Anxiety

Fear plays a huge part in the emotional pain of chronically ill
and disabled people. We are afraid of the process of our illness,
we are afraid of pain, we are afraid of increasing loss of control,
we are afraid of the outcome, and we are afraid of dying. Heart
patients, cancer patients, and patients with nervous system or
immune system disorders are all afraid of recurrences—we live
always with the knowledge that, no matter how well we feel at
breakfast, by lunchtime we may have felt something or noticed
something about the way our body moves, and we are sucked
into the obsessive fear of a recurrence. Add to this the fear many
of us have of the medical establishment. Our fear may be based
on mistrust due to past experiences; it may be based on a mature understanding that doctors are not shamans (priests who
use magic) and that most medicine is not miraculous. We are
afraid of our treatment and of side effects that can be painful
and debilitating. We have financial concerns which, as bills and
worries about insurance coverage mount, often become major
fears.

And we have fears relating to our families and friends. We are
afraid of how they see us, how they feel about us, and how our
condition affects their lives. Many people with degenerative illnesses spend many hours fearing the future of their loved ones
— afraid of having to use up family financial resources during
the course of their disease, afraid of how a spouse will support

and take care of the children as the illness gets worse, or afraid that friends will feel increasingly obligated to offer help.

Fear is a sneaky emotion. It creeps up and grabs us when we least expect it, such as when we are watching a glorious sunset following a thunderstorm, looking at a brilliant red hibiscus blossom against the snow falling outside the window, or enjoying a moment full of love and serenity at a Thanksgiving dinner. At times of normal activity, intense joy, or contentment, fear may whisper in our ear and the energy that was happiness may have to be used to put down fear, robbing our spirits.

Then there is anxiety, the way our minds protect us from fear. When we become too afraid of our fear, our minds often simply blank it out with the buzzing of anxiety or panic. And we can't function. The anxiety associated with fear can, in itself, become chronically disabling.

Yet fear can also bless us. When we recognize fear as a separate and manageable psychological response to emotional pain, we have the key which allows us to choose how we are going to respond to powerlessness, isolation, anger, grief, or any of the other pains that we experience in our illness or disability. We can choose fear, or we can replace it with hope and faith.

Isolation

The feeling of isolation is an emotional pain that can become overpowering. Whether we have a new illness or a long-term disability, we often feel alone and somehow outside of the "normal" world. We may feel alone, even among those who love and care for us. No one seems to really understand our feelings; we are different, and there is no way to wipe away that difference.

When a man sits in a wheelchair, or a woman shakes with cerebral palsy, their difference is obvious, and it is also apparent in the way they are treated by others. This treatment, in itself, can isolate them. Often, when obviously disabled people are in a group, either much self-conscious attention is given them, or they are benignly ignored.

People with conditions not obvious to an observer often feel isolated too. They feel helpless to explain themselves, or they spend emotional energy trying to pass as nondisabled.

A middle-aged woman, recently diagnosed with lung cancer, has lunch with a group of friends. When asked how things are in her life, she says, "Great, just great," and feels as alone as she has ever felt. An older man, athletic all of his life but now in an early stage of Parkinson's disease, avoids helping his hostess serve coffee because he can't trust himself to carry the cups. He excuses himself and goes into the bathroom, where he leans against the wall feeling alone and despairing.

The antidote for isolation is involvement with others. A person might wonder why the chronically ill and disabled don't resolve their loneliness by reaching out. There are many reasons. We don't reach out because we don't want pity. We don't reach out because we don't want to have to explain. We don't reach out because we don't want to appear weak, as if we can't keep a stiff upper lip, or cope. When we say, "I have lupus," or heart disease, or cancer, then we are identified as having lupus, or heart disease, or cancer, and that makes it more real. We can't fool ourselves into pretending for even a little while that the condition isn't really there. Finally, and perhaps most devastatingly, we don't reach out because we are ashamed.

Feelings of shame and isolation are wound together in a knotted mass. We may feel ashamed that we are different, that we aren't perfect, that perhaps somehow we are responsible for our condition. We may feel ashamed of our physical weakness, or feel we are grotesque, or think of ourselves as a source of contamination. Our feelings of shame may lead us to fears about how to present ourselves to others, which can lead to lowering self-esteem and increasing isolation.

When we use the Twelve Steps to help ourselves work through the pain of isolation, we may find a potential blessing in separation and aloneness. Isolation can give us the time to meet and come to understand our true selves—and to learn that we can survive. It also does us an immense favor. To relieve the pain of isolation, we are forced to reach out to others, to join the human community we all need to become spiritually whole.

Anger and Rage

We experience anger and rage in chronic illness and disability differently, depending on our personalities and upbringing.

When Marilyn describes her rage at her severe, disfiguring psoriasis (a chronic skin disease), she says, "Sure, I'm really angry about it all, but if I think about my anger it feels more like despair or pleading. When I talk about being angry there isn't much feeling in it. But if I think how the anger looks inside my head—it's just a flaming, rolling red mass."

This internal conflict seems to reflect what some of us may have learned about anger: we have it, but we shouldn't express it. Some people, on the other hand, have no difficulty feeling and expressing their anger, and they rage at their condition. "God! When I think about it I could kill!" is not an unusual reaction.

Anger and rage can rise out of different aspects of problems. Some of us get rageful because our bodies have betrayed us; others of us are rageful due to our sense of powerlessness. Some of us have much anger about the meaninglessness of our illness or at the person or situation we blame for bringing it on. Some people's anger comes from feelings of jealousy and resentment, or from a sense of being trapped, or from feeling caught in the spiral into recurrence.

We may get angry at a lot of different things: at God, nature, life, the world, medicines, doctors, treatments, hospitals, and even at family and friends for not understanding us or not responding exactly as we want them to at a certain moment. We may get angry when people make allowances for us or when they don't. We may rage at our caregivers, alienating them or turning them into martyrs. Or we may place our rage on other things: our children's behavior, other drivers, or politicians.

We might project our anger on others, believing they are angry with us for something we did or didn't do, or said or didn't say. Anger can become a tool of power when we feel powerless and can become a way that we manipulate others. Our rage can take the form of self-destructive behaviors such as drug abuse, suicide attempts, reckless driving, or perhaps it is just too much to deal with and we suppress it and become despondent or depressed.

The real power of rage and anger is that it has energy—lots and lots of energy. And the energy of rage can be useful if we turn it away from self-destruction and use its strength as an emotional basis for growth. Determination can grow from the energy of anger—determination to stretch our physical boundaries and determination to expand our spiritual selves. Much as a rocket needs the massive thrust of flaming energy for blast-off, the flaming energy of rage can propel us toward the heights of emotional wellness.

Blame and Ambiguity

Most of us certainly don't feel ambiguous about our illnesses or disabilities—we don't want them. But we have them and somehow have to make sense of them. Before we can accept or adapt to just about anything in our life, we have to be able to make sense out of it, we have to give it meaning. When we are struck with a chronic illness or become disabled, we feel a need to figure out why and what it means. To do this we need to decide who or what is responsible for our condition. Here is where blame enters. When something of little consequence happens to us we can place the responsibility for it without much emotion. But when the event is a very negative one we may respond with all kinds of painful emotions, and this can turn into blaming. The question becomes, "Whose fault is this?"

We may feel ambiguous about the answer. Do we blame fate, a doctor's misdiagnosis, faulty medical treatment, a gene, or another person who caused an accident? Do we put the blame on an external source? Or do we internalize it, shaming ourselves for what we did or what we didn't do to prevent whatever it is that hurts us? Blaming others often turns to open rage that moves into many areas of our lives; blaming ourselves often leads to self-hatred and depression.

No matter which direction we point the finger of blame, there is no peace for us, so some people try a different trick. They sidestep the issue of fault by redefining the condition, giving it meaning in a way that whoever is responsible doesn't matter.

The mother of a sixteen-year-old boy who, while drunk, drives into a ditch at 2:30 in the morning, breaking his neck and becoming quadriplegic, says, "He was driving home from a party at the church and swerved to avoid a young couple walking along the edge of the road."

She comes to believe that his accident occurred because of a self-sacrificing act on her son's part. The negative emotion is buried in a positive context, and she has peace without blame.

A woman who is diagnosed in her mid-thirties with multiple sclerosis says, "This must be God's way of telling me to reorganize the priorities in my life."

She no longer has to worry about whose fault her illness is. Whether or not we agree with this kind of mental gymnastics, this way of making sense of the situation does help us avoid ambiguity and relieves the pain associated with blaming.

Blame and ambiguity are particularly hard for those of us with illnesses that go into remission and then recur. Every time we have a remission, we wonder what we or someone else did that caused it. Then when a recurrence starts, many of us think, *What did I do to make it worse? Should I change my diet, vitamins, exercise, or medication?* We try harder and harder to figure it out, putting more and more pressure on ourselves, wondering *What is really wrong with me?*

New techniques of stress reduction, mental imagery, and positive thinking add another dimension to placing blame. It is very hard for people to understand that, while these techniques can be extremely beneficial in reducing the strain on our already overtaxed systems, they may make us better but are not often going to permanently cure us. A man with heart disease who spends time every day meditating and visualizing his heart as strong and healthy can bring down his blood pressure, perhaps reduce his medication, and feel much more serene. But he still is at above average risk of stroke or heart attack. And that is not his fault. His efforts have helped, but he is not to blame for the fact that he isn't cured.

Through dealing with ambiguity and blame we can begin to unravel the meaning of our illness or disability and work through much of the denial that keeps us stuck with our emotional pain. We can also learn to realistically assign responsibility, which helps us see our situation clearly: our minds become unclouded by blaming, and our spirits become free of confusion.

Jealousy

Envy, resentment, and jealousy are emotional pains that are very hard for us to separate from each other and very hard to eliminate. Our values and beliefs may be deeply rooted in competition, and often it is competition that is at the base of jealousy, envy, and resentment. To envy is to wish we had something that someone else has. To resent is to be angry and bitter because we don't have what someone else has. And to be jealous is to have feelings of anger, sometimes hatred, toward the person who has what we want. Because so much emphasis is placed on perfection, none of us escapes feelings of jealousy, envy, and resentment from time to time. But when we are struck with a chronic illness or disability these feelings can become a monumental influence in our lives.

We may be resentful because we are different, and we may envy and be jealous of people whose lives are not impaired by illness and disability—people who move and speak easily and don't live with fear about the betrayal of their bodies. We may envy what we see as the freedom of their lives.

A young girl in a wheelchair watches from her front porch as her neighborhood friends go off to the swimming pool, and she envies them—she is jealous of the other girls. She is concentrating on what others have. As she envies her friends she cannot appreciate her own skill with her flute; while her emotional energy is used for jealousy she forgets how hilarious she and those same girls got yesterday while they played Trivial Pursuit.

Jealousy keeps her focused on the impossible; she forgets her own potential.

Yet those of us who are cursed with jealousy can also experience its blessing. When we use the Twelve Steps and commit ourselves to release our jealousy, we can learn to stop comparing ourselves to others, and to value ourselves as incredibly wonderful, unique people, important and acceptable just as we are.

Grief

It is necessary and normal for us to experience grief with the onset of a disability or chronic illness. "Necessary and normal" doesn't lessen the pain; it simply says that we are going to grieve.

The woman who takes her stroke "like a brick" is hiding her grief—perhaps to take care of herself, perhaps to take care of those around her—and her attitude will limit her ability to truly come to peace with her condition.

After years spent working with terminally ill patients, Dr. Elisabeth Kübler-Ross described the grief process associated with death, and her work, *On Death and Dying,* is still considered the classic in the field. Now scholars have taught us that the grief process is associated with all loss, whether it is moving from one home to another, getting married or divorced, or becoming disabled or chronically ill.

All change involves loss, even happy change. When some of us are married we are happy to begin a new life with a beloved person; at the same time we may grieve the loss of our single life. If we have a second child, we may grieve the loss of the little family we have had until that time. And when we are disabled or develop a chronic illness, we may grieve for the person that we were, the life that we had been living, our changed relationships, or our lost future.

Some griefs are small, some are large, some almost overwhelm us—but whatever the degree, the process is the same. There are three phases of grief. First comes denial, shock, numbness, and disbelief.

Seventeen-year-old Jake has been in a hospital for three weeks. He is out of intensive care and recovering, but a diving accident has left him quadriplegic. Jake simply cannot believe that he will never walk again; he feels numb, not comprehending his situation. He will tell friends, "The doctors say this is permanent, but they don't know me!" His mother, Esther, can't believe it either. "I just don't seem to feel anything," she says.

People with illnesses or disabilities that aren't obvious often get stuck in this phase as they continually try to pass as "normal." The denial associated with passing as "normal" keeps them from moving on toward acceptance of their conditions.

The second phase of grief is one of intense emotional pain. Extreme mood swings, overwhelming sadness, raging grief, depression, lethargy, hyperactivity, regression to childlike helplessness, despair, guilt, and bargaining with doctors or God — all these are emotions and behaviors that can possess us.

And then there is our anger. We may be angry at everyone and everything. We may lash out toward others or turn anger inward on ourselves. This phase may last for a long time—the greater the loss, the less prepared for it we are, the more limited our options, and the longer it will continue. The danger is that we will get stuck in it.

While grief is normal, it is a process, and should be moved through—slowly, over a long period of time, with many regressions, but nevertheless with movement. But some people stop. They don't stop grieving—they just stop moving, and their grief becomes chronic. They continue to promise God that they will never smoke again if He will remove their lung cancer. They stay deeply depressed, refusing to do things to relieve their depression and using it as a way to manipulate those around them.

They refuse to care for their bodies, insisting that a caregiver feed and dress them. They wallow in guilt, and rage at the world.

Ultimately, most people with a stable disability or unremitting disease move beyond these first two phases of grief. But people with illnesses that have periods of remission and recurrence can have a great deal of trouble. Every time their illness retreats, hope springs up, and hope may beget denial. Then when, inevitably, illness recurs, the second phase of grief starts all over again. And they may be unable to move to the final phase.

In the last phase of grief we learn to let go of the past, and to accept ourselves as we are. We learn to live with our situation and to again look forward. Even people with terminal illness tell us that they can find acceptance, peace, and a sense of the future. Their future may be measured in only days or hours, but their eyes and emotions are in the present. They look forward to seeing friends and loved ones, perhaps to eating a special food or watching birds on a feeder. *Maybe this afternoon or tomorrow the narcissus will bloom,* they may tell themselves. Many of them envision an afterlife reflecting their religious beliefs and gain hope.

The blessing of grief is in its process. We are thrown into grieving, we feel its pain and agony, yet we finally can come to acceptance. To go through the grieving process can give us a deeply rooted faith that everything passes, that there is some way to deal with whatever we must deal with, and that we will come out into the light. Somehow, grief cleanses us; we are left ready to rebuild.

Exhaustion

Many of us with chronic illness or disability also suffer from chronic exhaustion. We can be overwhelmed by the physical barriers we face.

The sheer energy used by a stroke victim as she struggles with her walker to the bathroom; the sheer energy used by a paraplegic as he is lowered from his van, wheels across a sidewalk, and maneuvers to open a huge plate glass door;

27

*the sheer energy used by a man with Parkinson's as he nego-
tiates the stairs in his apartment house—it all results in
exhaustion, and it is a way of life.*

Add to this the energy sapped by the emotional pains, the
negative feelings that we live with. Even when we are experiencing the energy-renewing feelings of contentment, satisfaction, or
joy, we are always just a hairsbreadth away from fear, loneliness,
anger, and depression. It is no wonder we are tired.

It's hard to see how exhaustion can bless us. Like severe
depression, it leaves us drained, and passionless. But when we
feel empty and at the end of our rope, for most of us there is an
instinctive urge toward survival. Within our deepest core we
can find a way to connect with living. We may be physically and
emotionally tired, but spiritually we have strength that we can
use to help ourselves.

Breaking out of the Pain Cycle

These are some of the emotional pains that unite chronically
ill and disabled people. Unfortunately, many of our cultural beliefs and many of our religions don't necessarily help relieve the
pain. As young children we may have learned that "We will get
what we deserve in life," which for chronically ill or disabled
people translates into, "I must be pretty bad to have had this
happen to me." This can create guilt and lowered self-esteem.
We may be taught that "Suffering ennobles a person," meaning,
"I have to be a good sport about this, pretend that everything's
great, even though I hate it with all my heart." This can result
in suppression of our grief and not accepting ourselves. We may
be taught that "Everything that happens, happens for a purpose." Translation: "If this has happened to me, there must be a
reason and I've got to figure out what it is." This can mean
months, perhaps years, of fruitless struggle to find meaning in a
purposeless, life-diminishing event such as a motorcycle wreck
or swimming pool accident.

It would be wrong to say that chronically ill and disabled people are constantly experiencing, or being overwhelmed by, emotional pain. But it is a significant and crippling part of our lives. For many of us the unresolved anger, grief, and feelings of powerlessness keep us stuck in our spiritual development, cycling round and round rather than taking a straight path toward growth. In doing this, we increase the negative effects of our illness and the extent of our disability.

To break out of the cycle, we can work through our pain and replace it with determination, satisfaction, contentment, happiness, joy, and serenity. Although each of us brings a unique personality to this task, we can all reexamine our lives and our values. We can fight denial and accept the unacceptable. We can decide that our lives are worth living, even with the illness or disability that we suffer, and we can find spiritual meaning.

The Twelve Step program of A.A. gives us a map for our spiritual growth as chronically ill or disabled people. A.A. is built on the premise that alcoholism is a spiritual illness as well as a chronic, degenerative physical illness. The alcoholic has a chronic, spiritual illness focused around alcohol. Those of us who suffer chronic illness or disability have a spiritual illness too. Our spiritual illness has grown out of our emotional pain. This pain can keep us focused on our physical condition and stunt our spiritual growth. The Twelve Steps offer us a new way to live. They provide a way that we can turn the threat of our illness or disability into a challenge toward living the fullest life possible. In making them the pattern for our lives we can achieve a spiritual wellness that can become more important than our physical condition. We can find serenity and joy.

CHAPTER FOUR

THE TWELVE STEP JOURNEY

The Twelve Step program of A.A. provides a way of life that can relieve the emotional pain connected with chronic illness and disability and offers a design for reaching spiritual health. The emotional pain connected to our physical condition is destructive of our spirituality—it keeps us cycling around our illness or disability so we are unable to use emotional energy to grow in a more productive way. In this chapter we will learn how our emotional pain can be alleviated.

The Twelve Step journey is to be taken one day at a time and at a pace that is comfortable for you. The First Step is accepted and made a part of our lives—followed by the Second, Third, Fourth, and so on through the whole program. As we work a Step, we may have new insights about an earlier one, so we go back and think some more, making changes or additions to what we had done before. The objective is to continually deepen our understanding and to translate this understanding into the way we live our lives.

The Steps are not a test; speed, competitiveness, correctness, and perfection don't matter. The goal is our individual spiritual wellness. We reach this goal by feeding our spirits as we move from Step to Step, accepting ourselves and our lives, releasing our pain, and deepening our spiritual awareness. Most of us won't experience a spiritual awakening as a single inspirational event; instead, we have one small awakening after another, and they add up. This new philosophy and new way of life is not easily gained. It takes much patience, great effort, and tolerance for the times we slip back into old ways—remembering that old habits will fight hard to stay with us.

But the Twelve Steps can help us. They suggest humility, a willingness to face facts, a freedom from false pride, grandiosity, and arrogance. They suggest honesty, freedom from self-deception, trustworthiness in our thoughts and behaviors, sincerity in our desire to eliminate our pain, and a willingness to admit that we have been following an unhealthy path. They suggest faith and a belief in a Power whose will is greater than our own. We can draw strength from the Twelve Step program as it leads us to a spiritually fulfilled life. The Twelve Steps also suggest courage, the fortitude to endure the things we cannot change, and the appreciation of the ways we can change. Finally, they suggest service, reaching out to others who need and want the same kind of help that we have needed and wanted. When we can change our old ways of being, and carefully and consciously live as the Twelve Steps instruct, slowly, slowly our spirituality can be enriched, and we can become more than we have ever been.

What follows is a closer look at the suggested Twelve Steps of A.A., adapted for our condition of chronic illness or disability. After each Step is described, there are written and imagery exercises to help you better understand and practice the Step. Because of differing personalities, some people will prefer one method, some the other, some both, and some will make up a unique exercise to fit their own needs. It doesn't matter. Do whatever is comfortable for you, but try to do it.

The written exercise will be most helpful if you answer in as much detail as possible. Write on a separate sheet of paper and take as much time as you need—there are no "correct" answers and speed is irrelevant; it is the depth of response that matters.

The imagery exercises are designed to help you incorporate each Step into your life. They are not magic, but if practiced repeatedly and sincerely they are one of the most powerful tools we have to achieve spiritual growth. As Rokelle Lerner wrote in *Affirmations*, "Who (or what) you see in your imagination will always rule your world." Everyone images differently. Some people see pictures in their minds; some simply have sensations or feelings that represent to them the contents of the image. However it works for you, accept it. There are no right ways to do the imagery exercises—wherever your mind leads you is the most effective way to meet the subconscious part of yourself, to let it tell you what you already know but cannot reach. It is through your subconscious mind that you can get in touch with your Higher Power, and imaging allows that contact to be made without the interference of your conscious ego.

POWERLESS YET POWERFUL

Step One: We admitted we were powerless over chronic illness—our lives had become unmanageable. *

Step One asks us to admit that our chronic illness or disability causes us emotional pain, that we are powerless over this pain, and that we cannot control it, move away from it, or manage it. To most of us this is an appalling idea. We have struggled so hard with our condition that the last thing we want to admit is powerlessness over the pain it causes us. We spend much of our energy denying, pretending that our physical condition is what matters, and ignoring the fact that our emotional pain is a problem in itself.

Sarah, a 36-year-old wife and mother of two children, has recurrent breast cancer. "I work so hard at it. I use healing imagery, watch my diet like a hawk, do everything the doctors

---

*Adapted from the Twelve Steps of Alcoholics Anonymous, reprinted with permission of A.A. World Services, Inc., New York, N.Y. The original Twelve Steps of A.A. appear in Appendix Two.

suggest, exercise, almost kill myself trying to use positive thinking. I just can't believe that I don't have control over this disease! If I believed that, it would be like giving up, and giving up means dying."

Sarah defines her fears and anxieties as emotions "not to give in to" because then she might "give up" and die.

Brad is 50 and quite crippled. When he was 35 he was diagnosed with multiple sclerosis and has struggled daily to maintain all the physical function he could. Many, many times he yearned to give up, to stop working so hard for so little— just trying to hold back the onslaught of complete dysfunction. "But," he says, "if I hadn't done my damnedest to stay in control over this thing, I might be completely helpless by now."

Brad denies that emotional pain plays any part in his struggle.

Ella has had cerebral palsy since birth. Every day for 42 years she has fought to keep herself in control—to be as much like other women as she can. "Control, manage, control, manage, those two words hold the story of my life. They're what I know best in the world."

Ella can't describe serenity.

In many ways what these valiant people say is true. They *do* take responsibility for themselves, they *do* work at controlling their lives, they *do* constantly try to manage, and while they control and manage, they deny the importance of their emotional pain.

For those of us who live with physical illness or disability it is particularly hard to accept the idea of personal powerlessness. We are accustomed to working hard to deal with a physical condition that has been handed to us by fate, and most of us take full, active responsibility for our lives. We look strong, we cope, but we can't fool our psyches: our emotional pain does not go away. Instead, it remains unmanageable. It stays with us despite our best efforts and for just one reason: We continue to fight, deny, and attempt to overcome our powerlessness in the face of our chronic illness or disability. We keep trying to manage the unmanageable and the feelings of helplessness, hopelessness, rage, panic, despair, fear, anxiety, jealousy, and grief continue.

The First Step is the foundation of the A.A. recovery program. It is not meant as a Step in which we judge ourselves, but as an opportunity to objectively observe our behavior and admit that we cannot continue alone, that we need help. Admitting this need for help is a way of surrendering, and surrendering breaks through our denial and lets us be honest with ourselves. When we choose to surrender, to let go, we have, in a way, chosen to be in control of not being in control.

To Surrender Is to Win

For our logical minds, this may be a hard concept to understand. Perhaps it will help to look at the postures of t'ai chi, the ancient Chinese ritual dance of life.

If we study t'ai chi, we find that the posture for Strength is to stand erect, arms extended straight out to the side from the shoulders, palms turned upward, legs straight, and feet planted firmly on the ground. The entire body is held in rigid control, pressing upward as if to support an immense load of weight bearing down on it, fully engaged with external pressure. This forced, stress-filled pose begins the dance, which then flows into the posture of Power.

In Power, the legs remain straight, feet solidly grounded, but the arms and shoulders curve in. The head drops to the chest, and the entire upper body is rounded, pulled in, curved down toward the abdomen. To us in the Western world this may look like a pose of abject surrender, but to the Chinese it represents the gathering in, the protection of energy within the very center of the body. This is Power because the energy is carried within. There is disengagement with external stress, and the body presents a form that the pressures of the world can pour over, slide down, and flow away from. Strength uses up our energy, while Power conserves and increases it.

The First Step asks us to surrender our Strength and choose a concept of Power much like the t'ai chi. It asks us to give up our straining grit-our-teeth, clench-our-jaw efforts to control the world around us and to carry its weight on our shoulders. Instead, it suggests we give up our struggles to manage, to bend down and gather in our energy, and to hold it within ourselves.

As we work the First Step we are asked to put aside the pride that has taken so much of our energy. We are asked to become humble. Humility does not mean giving up our selfhood, nor does it mean to bow down. Humility is about equality and place. When we are humble we may be less powerful, but we are not less important. People are certainly humble before, and have less power than, nature. But without people, nature is not complete. To become humble is to accept our place, without arrogance or grandiosity, in the overall scheme of life. Though the degrees of power we have may differ, everyone and everything is important and is equally necessary in making and maintaining the whole.

The First Step also asks that we admit our obsessive need to control and manage. It asks that we accept our powerlessness over our emotional pain. It tells us that our spiritual journey to serenity begins with surrender. In the past, the satisfaction we experienced when we had everything under control might have been called a kind of serenity. But that serenity could be instantly threatened—at any moment we could lose control. The serenity we experience when we give up our attempts to maintain everlasting control, when we surrender to our powerlessness, can never be threatened: we have no control to lose.

To Surrender Is Not to Quit

"Surrender" is a frightening word to many of us. We surrender in wartime to our enemies. We surrender something when we give it up to someone else. And we surrender when we quit. As very young children we may be taught that good guys win and losers surrender—so, by the definition we understand, surrenderers are quitters and losers. We sometimes hear that we surrender in love, but even then surrendering has an overtone of weakness.

Sarah believes that if she surrenders she will die. Brad thinks surrender would mean total helplessness, and Ella has had a life so full of holding on to control that the concept of surrender is as foreign to her as the world of science fiction. But if we think about it there are wonderful aspects to surrender. If we surrender to our sense of powerlessness, we have a potential for getting real help and nurturing.

If Sarah surrenders the outcome of her condition, she can be more realistic in expending her limited energy and ask those who love her to support her in ways that can make her life less frantic and more meaningful. Brad can gain relief from putting down the impossible burden that he has tried to carry alone. He can feel closer to his wife, more as though she were a part of his true reality, and accept her help. Finally, Ella can find relief from the pressure of trying to belong that has plagued and narrowed her life. In surrender, she can learn how serenity feels.

Surrender does not mean giving up responsibility for our actions or our emotional pain. It does mean understanding and accepting the fact that we cannot control the outcome of our condition and are powerless over the pain that it brings us. When we acknowledge this our healing begins. The emotional energy that has been bound in pain is released, and we can use it for intimacy, love, and creativity. In our surrender to powerlessness, we find energy for the powerful emotions that can lead us to spiritual health.

Step One: Written Exercise

1. When you look back on your life, how important has control been to you in relation to your chronic illness or disability?

2. What difficulties are you having in (a) recognizing your powerlessness over the emotional pain attached to your illness or disability and (b) in recognizing that your life has become unmanageable?

3. How is your emotional pain affecting your current life?

4. Which of the emotional pains listed in this chapter are the most unmanageable for you, and which of them would you like most to be free of?

5. How do you define humility? What are its positives and negatives?

6. How do you define surrender? What are its positives and negatives?

7. If you are relieved of your emotional pain, how can this change your life?

Step One: Imagery Exercise

Close your eyes and allow an image of yourself to come into your mind. Picture yourself walking in the woods. You are carrying a heavy packsack that strains at its seams. Try to imagine this packsack in detail—its color, size, how it fits on your back. Does it have a frame? Or is it supported by your neck and shoulders alone? If you have never carried a pack, just imagine what it looks like and how it feels to support its weight on your back.

Imagine that this pack carries everything you need to control all of the pain, all of the power you try to maintain, and all of the managing skills that you've worked so hard for. As you keep walking through the woods, you stumble every now and then over rocks or exposed roots in the path. You have to keep your head down—pulling forward in order to support the weight on your back. Feel the strain in your neck and see the path under your feet. You can't look upward, or even very far forward, because that would throw you off balance and you might fall.

Now imagine that the path ends at the edge of a meadow. With your peripheral vision you can just barely see long green grass, bending in the light breeze. Blue forget-me-nots and white daisies are in bloom. Feel yourself standing on the edge of this meadow, yearning to run free, or to lie down in the fragrant grass and rest with the sun pouring its energy into you. But to do this, you must first put down your pack; you can neither run nor rest while carrying this load.

Now do it. Swing the pack off of your shoulders and let it drop to the ground. Hear the crunching sound it makes as it hits the ground. Take a moment to enjoy the feeling of lightness and relief. Straighten up, stand there, and savor the release. You begin to move away from the pack; it lies there at the edge of the meadow and soon you can't see it anymore. Allow yourself to feel the freedom. It's all right, you don't have to feel guilty or afraid, just relish the lightness. You've left your need to control, to manage, in that pack; now you are powerless and free, powerless and full of a feeling of confidence, comfort, and serenity.

Just for now, don't think about what happens to your power, who gets it or where it goes. As a controller you are always thinking ahead, straining to meet the future before its time, but now you must learn to take one step at a time. Simply feel the freedom that comes with putting down your load. PERIOD. Feel the freedom and get used to it—it's the First Step.

Now, open your eyes and resume your life. During the day stop for a moment now and then. Remember the feeling of freedom you had when you put down the pack and admitted you were powerless by dropping all your efforts at control.

FINDING OUR POWER SOURCE

Step Two: Came to believe that a Power greater than ourselves could restore us to sanity.

The Twelve Step program first requires that we admit our powerlessness, and change our controlling, managing, manipulative behaviors. Then it asks that we accept the unconditional existence of a spiritual force, a Power greater than ourselves, that we are willing to believe can heal our emotional pain. The First Step suggests the change we need to make in our lives; the Second Step lays the spiritual basis for the program.

Came to believe that a Power greater than ourselves . . .

This phrase often causes confusion, misunderstanding, and outright rejection of the Twelve Step program. Many, many people hear it and say, "I just cannot believe in God." They don't understand that neither God nor religion is an issue. What is the issue is the existence of some Power outside of ourselves that has more control over our lives than we do.

Many of us who struggle with chronic illness or disability have come to believe in self-sufficiency. As a consequence we may have become isolated; our self-sufficiency has created barriers both between ourselves and other people and ourselves and a Higher Power. Even for those of us who believe in a traditional God, it may be hard to place Him in our lives. He certainly hasn't taken away our condition nor made clear why we must suffer. Some of us are agnostics, some atheists. Many of us may have never taken the time or made the effort to develop our own spiritual philosophy. To seriously consider what we believe about life, about living, about how the universe is formed and directed, is time consuming and hard work. Other things are more pressing; the living of life often takes precedence over the contemplation of it.

We tend to confuse religion with spirituality, believing that if we think about "spiritual" things then we must somehow tie them in with "religious" belief. When we try to understand the meaning of "Came to believe that a Power greater than ourselves," what we need to do first is to separate religion and spirituality. The Twelve Steps is a spiritual program, not a religious one. When we talk about spirituality, we are talking about the spirit of life. This spirit is made up of the force that makes life happen together with our belief in its power. For religious people, this life force may be God. For people who do not have traditional religious beliefs, it may not be.

Spirituality is a great enigma. We cannot see it, touch it, or measure it. Yet, it has existed throughout history, across many different systems of thought. Humankind has probably always recognized and expressed spirituality.

Developing Our Spirituality

Neither religious nor scientific thinkers have ever agreed about what spirituality is or where it is located. Most of us are not philosophers; we can't argue the fine points of science and spiritual or religious doctrine. But we can think through a spiritual philosophy for ourselves. While our personal philosophy may change and deepen over time, the important thing for us to do now is to begin. And that is what the Second Step asks us to do.

Our willingness to surrender and believe in the process of the Twelve Steps helps us to let go of our self-will. When this happens, a block is removed and our subconscious becomes much more available to us. It may give us messages in dreams and odd, fleeting thoughts. Strange coincidences may occur and we may recognize signs of a presence that we have been unaware of until now. Slowly the idea of a "Power greater than ourselves" can become easier to grasp and more acceptable to us. As we stop trying to singlehandedly manage both our chronic illness or disability and the emotional pain that comes with it, we begin to consider that perhaps a Higher Power can help us.

There are no rules for the form our individual Higher Power will take. It can be whoever or whatever we choose. Some choose God as they understand Him or Her. Some choose an image that occurs in their mind. Some choose human love, nature, or the universe. Some choose the Twelve Step program itself. The form simply does not matter; what matters is belief that the Power exists and is greater than we are.

Rhoda has kidney disease and her life is limited by dialysis and the other protocols that go with her condition. She is Jewish, but left the practice of Judaism several years before she married a man with no professed religious belief. Rhoda's

41

Higher Power is an oak tree. "I know that sounds really silly, but when I look at a tree, particularly an oak tree, I know that there is something that controls our universe. When I call on my Higher Power I also have some stirrings of old stuff, from back in the days when I was a practicing Jew. But I'm not ready to deal with that now, and that wonderful oak tree does the job."

Judy, who has had two mastectomies, says, "After years and years of thinking I had no religious belief left from my childhood, I've found that my Higher Power is God—and He's the God that I knew from Sunday school. I feel as though I've come home."

Dan has been an atheist all of his life, just like his father. Also, just like his father, he has severe heart disease. Dan sees the Twelve Step program as his Higher Power. "It isn't the people in the program that I think of as my Higher Power, although they're a terrific support. But it's the way the program is a representation of how all of us struggle, of our combined spiritual strength, and the caring for each other— that's what helps me. There's a lot to this program. It can fit anyone. You can take what you want and leave the rest."

Meg was raised in a strict Catholic home. It has been fifteen years since she was blinded by a freak accident in her mid-twenties. "I had a really hard time with this whole Higher Power idea. The God I had always known was a strict God, with rules and regulations that wouldn't quit. He was also vengeful; I could never make a mistake or He might send me to hell. I never felt that I could ask Him for anything because there was no way I was good enough to deserve His help or consideration. So when I began to think about a 'Power greater than myself' I went back and reinvented God. It was terribly hard and took a long time. But I've done it! Now I know that my God is an all-loving Father. I asked myself how it would feel to have a father that just loved me, no matter what I did. And you can't imagine the peace and freedom I feel now."

Jane is a woman in her mid-sixties, quite disabled by rheumatoid arthritis. She found her Higher Power by asking it to appear in her imagination—and it did. "For me, it's a huge white light. It is made up of all of the energy from all living things and that includes inanimate objects like rocks too. They live, just in a different way. Anyhow, all of this energy is combined in a huge pool and it's there for the asking, for anyone. The wonder of it is that not only do we use it when we need to, but our very being puts more energy back into that pool so it can never run out."

. . . could restore us to sanity.

Is the Second Step calling us insane? Is it saying that our unhealthy attitudes and behavior, our emotional pain, is a kind of insanity? In a way it is, and perhaps that's right. If we were completely rational observers, objectively evaluating someone who thinks, feels, and acts as we do, many of those thoughts, emotions, and actions would seem irrational. What this Step is really saying is that we can come to believe that a Power greater than ourselves can help us release our irrationality and lead us to spiritual fulfillment. This is the act of faith suggested by the Second Step.

There seem to be five major factors involved in our spiritual fulfillment—strength, humility, understanding, emotional stability, and peace of mind. Let's look closer at them.

Spiritual strength develops from our recognition of a Higher Power and our faith in its healing. It also develops from thinking through a personal spiritual philosophy.

We find humility when we follow the Twelve Step program, give up our obsession with control and management, and truly accept our equality as human beings.

Understanding comes when we break through denial and self-absorption and realize that others struggle as we do.

Giving up our focus on our condition, and allowing ourselves to accept the love, care, and support of our Higher Power and the community of Twelve Step followers can bring us emotional stability.

And surrendering to powerlessness over our condition and emotional pain, together with faith in the healing potential of our Higher Power, can give us peace of mind.

Perhaps when we think of spiritual fulfillment it is more useful to think of spiritual evolution. To evolve means to change, unfold, become more complex, and be more than we have been in the past. It means to develop against the forces of habit and inertia, to extend ourselves beyond wherever we think we are able to go. It means to choose the force within us that pushes us toward the difficult path of growth, and to transcend our chronic illness or disability and our emotional pain.

As our Higher Power becomes more a part of our lives, we can become more spiritually fulfilled. We can come to accept, respect, and love ourselves as we are without qualification. We can nurture ourselves and enrich the lives of others.

Now working the Twelve Steps, Meg says, "I don't really understand much of the philosophical talk, but what I do know is that I feel better than I have since I can remember. I'm not so angry, not so scared, and having a Higher Power I feel more in place."

No matter what feelings or emotional pain we are dealing with, the fact is that looking at reality, admitting our powerlessness over the situation, and being supported by a loving, caring Power greater than ourselves can remove our emotional pain— without relieving the illness or disability. Rhoda's oak tree, Meg or Judy's God, Dan's Twelve Steps, or Jane's white light: any of these very individual Higher Powers can be the source of removing emotional pain. The form doesn't matter, as long as it is ours, and as long as we believe in it.

Step Two is often referred to as the "Hope Step." It tells us that there is help available and that we can receive it if we come to believe. There is a way out, a way so difficult and so easy— to let go of our need to control both our condition and our emotions, and to accept our Higher Power and to ask it to help. We no longer need to struggle alone.

Step Two: Written Exercise

1. What fears or other roadblocks stand between you and your acceptance of a Higher Power?

2. What differences do you see between religion and spirituality?

3. If you decide to accept the existence of a Power greater than yourself, how do you think your life will change? List specific examples.

4. Describe how your self-will and self-absorption can block your acceptance of a Higher Power.

5. How does your childhood experience of religion and spirituality (the way your family taught you) influence the way you believe today? How does it help you? How does this experience get in your way?

6. What does the statement "The Twelve Steps have a spiritual foundation" mean to you?

7. How could a Power greater than yourself remove your emotional pain? Choose a specific painful emotion and imagine how this would work.

Step Two: Imagery Exercise

Close your eyes and imagine yourself alone somewhere—a neutral place, not wonderful and not frightening. Very carefully look at yourself, taking time to see your illness or disability exactly as it is and feel the emotional pains that go along with it. The pains may be a mishmash of nonspecific feelings, or they may be very clear, negative emotions. Just see yourself as you truly are and let the feelings wash over you.

Now ask your Higher Power to join you. Look at Him or Her or It, whatever it is for you, and experience how you feel when you can see It or sense Its presence.

Now ask this Higher Power to help your painful feelings go away. Wait, be still, and see what happens. Perhaps you will feel relief, freedom, or gratitude, or maybe you will feel very little change. Whatever happens is all right—this exercise works differently for everyone. Your Higher Power is yours alone and will help you in its own special way.

Now open your eyes. You can repeat this exercise daily, maybe even several times a day. Allow time, and you can experience a change in your feelings and a lessening in your emotional pain.

CHAPTER FIVE

GAINING STRENGTH THROUGH NEW BELIEFS

Steps One and Two are *thinking* Steps; Step Three calls for *action*. As we work through the first two Steps, we begin to develop a personal philosophy—we make a commitment to connect with our own spiritual force. In Step Three, our commitment is tested as we must make an active decision to turn our wills and lives over to this nebulous force outside of ourselves. For many of us this is even more difficult than the first Steps. It calls for active surrender, and as chronically ill or disabled people we are accustomed to trusting our own will, not surrendering to the will of others. When we are struggling with this idea it helps to remember that we haven't done such a good job of managing up to this point; painful feelings and destructive emotions still make up a good part of our lives.

POWER AT OUR FINGERTIPS

Step Three: *Made a decision to turn our will and our lives over to the care of God* as we understood Him.

In the first three Steps we lay the groundwork for our entire recovery program—Steps Four through Twelve build on this foundation. For this reason it is crucial for us to feel comfortable with the first three Steps, to feel truly able to carry out all that they ask. Take your time and review as much as necessary. There is no hurry. What is important is that we understand the ideas and accept the concepts. Rokelle Lerner's book, *Affirmations*, has a quote that may be particularly helpful when working the Third Step:

> I feel no fear of new beliefs today. I see that changing my beliefs helps me release old patterns of behavior. . . . Today I give my strength and power to new beliefs.

Made a decision to turn our will and our lives over . . .

To "make a decision" is clear-cut and easy to understand. But what about "to turn over"? Just what does this mean? For some people working the Third Step it means exactly what it says — to give away, to no longer have control over, to put whatever it is in someone else's hands.

Meg believes that from the time she "turned it over," God took control of her life. She came to believe that He has a purpose for whatever happens to her and is always with her. God is Meg's active partner in every facet of her life. She truly believes "Thy will be done."

For Jane, "turning it over" is a more abstract concept. She believes that "to turn over" means to ask for support from her outside force, her White Light. It also means to present the Light with her concerns and to live by the ideals she believes it represents. Meg's life is guided by God's words from the *Bible,* while Jane's ideals have been developed as she worked out a personal philosophy that includes her White Light. The relationships are different, but both women are equally dedicated to the process. Although Meg and Jane have slightly different belief systems, their underlying faith is the same. They understand that they are no longer operating alone—they have asked someone or something else to be the overlying power and influence in their lives.

The Third Step asks for our will and our lives. This could be a frightening idea, as if there would be nothing left of us, as if "our will and our lives" are no longer our own. And in a way this is true. Making a decision to turn over our will and our lives means that we no longer have sole control over ourselves. There is an outside force that we have committed to follow. But this does not mean that we give up and become passive.

To the contrary, most of us find that when we decide to turn our will and our lives over to a Power greater than ourselves, we are freed to become more active than we have been in the past. The pressure is off; we aren't going it alone. We have lots of emotional energy previously tied up in managing and controlling that's now free for other uses. We can take realistic responsibility for our choices, our actions, our feelings, and the principles and values by which we live. We can give up our willfulness as we search for beliefs and behaviors that reflect the will of our Higher Power. We can work at our lives in a way that represents the ideals of God, or Light, the Twelve Step program, or however we interpret our Higher Power. We can surrender the outcome, but retain responsibility in our lives. An A.A. saying very appropriate for the Third Step is, "When you're in a boat and a storm comes up, pray to God, but row toward shore."

When we first begin to turn over our will and lives, it may be confusing and hard to do. As chronically ill or disabled people, we may have a hard time seeing how all of this relates to our condition. Do we stop being actively involved in our own care? Of course not. In reality, we may become even more active in our role with doctors, therapists, and treatment, and more creative in the management of our disabilities. But our activity is different, because, as we become deeply involved with our Higher Power, the emotional pain that has stood in our way begins to decrease.

Dan talks about how his relationship with his doctor has changed since he began to work the Twelve Steps. "In the beginning," he says, "I was so angry, just full of rage, and I didn't trust anybody—least of all the guy that was making me face up to my problem. Then as I got involved with the Twelve Steps I got much less angry and my defensiveness went away. I felt much more confident with him [the doctor], and I could get my point across without the whole scene falling apart," Dan says. "When things got better and we began to have decent conversations, he thought they were just between us—if only he knew, I had the whole blasted Twelve Step program with me every time."

. . . to the care . . .

The Third Step tells us that we should turn over our will and our lives to the "care" of, and "care" is a wonderful word. It means to be nurtured, guided, inspired, supported, helped, and relieved of our emotional pain. "Care" means to be unquestioningly and unequivocally nurtured. The very word tells us that our Higher Power is benevolent, not vengeful.

When we are disabled or become seriously ill, the deepest and most immediate feeling we have is screaming, raging emotional pain. The small child that lives at our very core cries out for help to be taken care of, but no one hears. We try not to listen, and there is no comfort for that small child within. Yet, miraculously, when we take the Third Step the child begins to be comforted—our Higher Power hears and provides care. This becomes an unceasing process. Whether it is the small child within us who needs comforting, or ourselves who need help and support, the caring is there.

. . . of God as we understood Him.

To whom or what do we turn over our will and our lives? Step Two gave us an idea or an image of our personal Higher Power. In Step Three we begin to deepen that relationship. As we work to turn over our will and lives, we come to know our Higher Power. We need to ask for direction so we can discover by what values and principles we should live. We need to turn to our Higher Power for support, to have Its caring begin to remove our pain. We can learn to talk with our Higher Power, and, over time, this becomes less a self-conscious act and more a natural part of life. When we have questions about a decision or a course of action, we ask our Higher Power for direction. When we need help or support, we ask. When we need to be relieved of pain, we ask. We learn to ask and then to be still and wait for the response. If we are still, if we are patient, if we believe, the response will come. There are sayings that can help us keep the faith.

- Turn it over to the Program.
- Release it to the Light.
- Let go, let God.

When we finish the first three Steps, we have laid the foundation for the rest of our Twelve Step work. It's a turning point. Here are three short studies of how this first part of the program has worked for three very different people: Meg, Jane, and Dan.

Meg's Story

The car accident that blinded Meg at age twenty-six also left her depressed.

I couldn't, or wouldn't even try to do all the retraining and therapy that is provided for blinded people. I'd had two beers that night and was convinced that the whole thing was my own fault. I was ashamed. I felt like I was no good to anyone, like my whole life was over. Actually, I wanted to die—I don't know why I didn't. One of my therapists talked to me about religion, getting help from God, but the only God I understood would have blamed me just the way I blamed myself—so that idea was worse than useless.

After two years Meg's depression lifted enough so that she could live alone, keep a job, and take care of herself, but she remained isolated, living a much more limited life than her blindness required. Also, she was crippled by anxiety.

Then a woman at work suggested that I go with her to Al-Anon. She was kind. She said that if she could learn to live with an alcoholic husband, I should be able to learn to live with blindness. And at Al-Anon this tremendous thing happened—I got the chance to create my own Higher Power. It was okay to make up whatever kind of Power greater than myself I wanted to. So I made up my own God. I made Him to be just what I wanted, the perfect, loving Father. I turned myself over to Him and He's involved in my whole life. All I have to do is say "help" and He's there. All my fear and anxiety and depression are gone. I didn't think you could be blind and be normal, but I am.

Jane's Story

Jane, who is disabled with rheumatoid arthritis, tells how the program worked for her.

I've had this disease most of my adult life—sometimes it's worse, sometimes it goes into remission, but the trend is always down, and it always will be. Now, as I'm getting older, I'm really pretty disabled. Over the years I think my main reaction has been being discouraged from the never-ending struggle to control something I couldn't—that's real powerlessness. I've had lots of fear about what I'd be like in the end, and how soon I'd get that way. I've had lots of times you might call despairing, but I've always, always had to seem "up" and show that I could cope. And I always knew, inside of me, that nobody understood—that's real loneliness. Then I'd go into remission and hope would spring up, but there was always fear with it—like when would the other shoe drop again?

Over the years Jane tried many different kinds of help such as therapists and Eastern and Western religions. All helped for a little while, but nothing lasted. Jane drifted. Her spiritual life had no direction.

I got into pills, painkillers. It was a mess, and I ended up in A.A. I worked at it, just the way I'd worked at things in the past, but at that point in my life, after all that I'd been through, I didn't expect much. But there was this idea of my own Higher Power. I really did find this tremendous White Light inside of myself, and I really did turn myself over to it. What did I have to lose? And changes started, and they held. I'm convinced they held because my Light is really never-ending, and it fills me with its energy, and my exhaustion lifts. My grandmother used to talk about seeing the light. I guess this is it.

Dan's Story

When Dan's heart disease was diagnosed he was furious. Threatened by the possibility of a shortened life, he raged at the limitations his doctor put on him. He had to quit smoking, lose 30 pounds, stop eating hamburgers, fried potatoes, and ice cream. And walk a mile a day? He was a busy man—where in hell could he find time? Dan was in a box: he could change his ways or he could die—and he didn't want to do either one. So he raged, and he blamed, and he lashed out at his family, friends, and doctor. And, often, when he least expected it, fear would come and he'd break out in a cold sweat and his hands would shake.

Then Dan's brother-in-law, a recovering alcoholic, suggested Dan go with him to an A.A. meeting. When Dan yelled that A.A. stuff is "religious pap," his brother-in-law yelled back, "Just give it a try. What have you got to lose?"

What hooked me was the calmness of the meetings. People were intimate yet almost impersonal about it—I'd never seen anything like it. God was irrelevant to me, so the program itself became my Higher Power. Now my life is very, very different. The doctor claims my blood pressure's down because of diet and exercise and medication, but I know that would never have done it alone. It's the program that's taken away my rage and fear. The only medicine for those was what you might call "hanging out with my Higher Power."

The Little Red Book tells us that, as a result of Step Three, five things can happen:

1. we surrender our self-centeredness;
2. we relax;

3. we avoid confusing the spiritual growth of the Twelve Step program with religion;
4. we do not try to define God; and
5. we recognize and attempt to develop our spiritual possibilities.

In addition, as we work Step Three we may begin to experience oneness with our Higher Power, and that can have great value for us. As Judith Viorst writes in her book, *Necessary Losses*, that "experience of oneness can give us a respite from the solitude of separateness. And experiences of oneness can help us transcend our former limits, can help us grow."

Step Three: Written Exercise

1. How did working the First and Second Steps get you ready for Step Three?

2. List your blocks to turning over your will and life to your Higher Power—then rank them in order of how important they are to you.

3. Take the blocks you listed and write what's positive and negative about each one.

4. What do you think the outcome of turning your life and will over to a Higher Power would be?

5. How would you explain the statement that becoming dependent on your Higher Power is really a way of becoming free?

6. What do you think is meant by the statement, "Even if your ideas of your Higher Power are not clear, that's all right. What's necessary is that you believe in the process."

Step Three: Imagery Exercise

Close your eyes and imagine that you are alone, surrounded by some kind of barrier—a fence, a wall, a sheet of rigid plastic, glass panels like a greenhouse, whatever comes into your mind. The barrier is there because you, alone, have your disability or illness. You can't get out from behind it, and no one else can get in. Allow yourself to feel all the feelings you have about being alone, separated, and surrounded. Take time and let the feelings come, even the ones you almost never let yourself feel. Just for this moment it's safe to let them be there.

Now ask your Higher Power to come to you. Ask it to help you. Allow yourself to feel surrounded by the caring your Higher Power gives you. Perhaps it holds you in its arms, perhaps it simply contains you in its light and warmth. Whatever form the care takes, it is yours.

Now, taking your caring Higher Power with you, walk through the barrier that separates you from the world. Notice what happens to it as you pass through it. Notice the feeling you have as you get beyond it. Hold the feeling.

Now open your eyes. Quietly sit and hold the feeling of caring you received from your Higher Power and the strength you felt as you moved through the barrier. Carry this feeling with you as you return to your normal daily activities.

CHAPTER SIX

TAKING AN INVENTORY

Step Four: Made a searching and fearless moral inventory of ourselves.

Our purpose in working the Fourth Step is to expose harmful emotions and character traits and to change them in a way that ensures our spiritual development. In the first two Steps we have admitted that we need help and that there is a Power greater than ourselves available to help us. With the Third Step we turned our will and our lives over to that Higher Power.

But these three Steps are only the beginning of our journey toward spiritual fulfillment. Alone, they aren't enough. We are still insulated from the serenity and peace we search for. We may be trapped in our self-centeredness, false pride, and dishonesty. Our concern with our physical problems, our emotional pain, and our denial may have interfered with our mental powers. It may have lowered our physical resistance and in many cases brought about irrational thoughts and behaviors.

All of this can result in extreme mental and physical hardship for us, and anxiety and suffering for others. And our lives will not improve until we deal with the negatives that inhibit our growth: the powerlessness, fear and anxiety, isolation and shame, anger and rage, blame and ambiguity, jealousy, grief, and exhaustion.

The main roadblock that stands in our way is denial. For those of us with chronic illness or disability, denial is one of our most effective survival techniques, protecting us from more emotional pain than we can tolerate. But while denial drives our pain out of consciousness, it cannot erase that pain from our unconscious mind. The paradox is that while denial protects us from conscious hurt, it also keeps us from finding, facing, and ultimately releasing our negative emotions. In other words, our protector keeps us from the self-awareness that is the key to spiritual growth.

To defeat denial, we must find a way to recognize, meet, and understand that which is denied, in this case our emotional pain. We do this by first accepting our pain, then coming to understand what it means to us, and receiving the help of our Higher Power. The objective of the Fourth Step is to overcome denial and become clearly aware of our emotions and behaviors. Then we will be able to release our pain and use the energy it consumed for positive, spirit-enhancing changes.

Finding and Facing Our Pain

As we begin the Fourth Step it is helpful to think about the many, varied personalities we bring to it. Some of us are fairly flexible; it's quite easy for us to accept and assimilate new or different ideas. Some of us have personalities that are more set: it is harder, or takes longer, for us to incorporate changes in thinking. Some of us are what psychologists call "concrete" thinkers: we define things in terms of black and white, good and bad, right and wrong. Some of us think more abstractly: our view of things is more complicated. Some of us are older, with more life experience, some younger, with less living behind us. And some of us are fortunate to be blessed with high self-esteem, while others are less sure of their personal worth.

Having one or another kind of personality pattern is neither good nor bad. Such patterns are descriptions, not judgments. But each of us *does* have particular characteristics and, as a beginning of the Fourth Step, it is helpful to take an honest look at how our personalities are organized. Realistic acceptance of how our mind works will start to break down our denial and open the way to true self-awareness.

When we became ill or disabled, we each had a personality with which we met our situation, and we each bring our unique personality to the Twelve Step program. To a great degree, these individual personality patterns will decide how we engage in our spiritual journey. They will determine which of us are more controlled by rage and which by despair. They will decide which of us more easily overcomes feelings of powerlessness and which are locked in a seemingly unbreakable cycle of grief. But no matter who we are, or how we think, the process will work. The crucial thing is to find and face our negative attitudes, our "character defects," and our pain, to commit ourselves to exposing them, and to accept the help of our Higher Power.

"What do you mean by 'find my pain'?" Meg asks. "Obviously I feel it or I wouldn't try so hard to overcome it."

We *do* often feel the emotional pain attached to our condition. The very intensity of our need to manage it is a measure of our need to deny it. And our need to deny it comes from fear. We are afraid that if we look at it, if we allow ourselves to experience it, it will be more real, it will become worse. The truth is that rarely in life can something be made worse by accepting its existence; rather, accepting its reality is the *only* way to begin to work through, or release, or change the situation or emotion. Unfortunately, what we often do is to look at the painful event or feeling and then quickly shy away from it because we are so afraid of it. Then we become afraid of not only the pain but also the fear. The cycle deepens and our protective denial builds. But working the Fourth Step can change this.

What follows in Chapter Seven is an inventory of the major emotional pains connected with our chronic illnesses or disabilities. The inventory includes two exercises, one written and one imagery, which can be used with each emotion discussed. The exercises, designed to increase self-awareness, are an important part of our work on the Fourth Step. The objective is to look at a certain pain, become familiar with it, and, consequently, reduce our fear of it. Ultimately, in Step Seven, we will ask our Higher Power to help to free us from our self-destructive behaviors and from the pain. But now our job is to remove it from the dark places where it lives and bring it into the full light of familiarity.

CHAPTER SEVEN

PAIN TO BE FOUND AND FACED

Powerlessness

"I picture myself as a broken leaf on a fast running stream, twirling around, being sucked under and then pulled back up to the surface," a young woman with multiple sclerosis says. "I am completely at the mercy of the water." A young man, quadriplegic, will spend his lifetime dependent on the care of others for his survival. An older woman with moderate heart disease can easily care for herself and can do many things to slow down the progression of her illness.

The degree of impairment is very different for these people, yet each knows that the results of their disease is not within the limits of their control; they all suffer from feelings of powerlessness.

Powerlessness is a strong, debilitating, natural response to chronic illness or disability. We feel powerless because we are powerless—powerless to make our condition go away, powerless to be "normal," powerless over whatever has happened to our bodies, powerless over the final outcome. This can lead to many other feelings—rage, panic, despair, lack of self-worth, anxiety, and on and on. And the behaviors that can grow out of our feelings of powerlessness are unhealthy and self-destructive: manipulation, passive aggression, helplessness, lashing out at those around us, isolation of ourselves, expectation of failure, just plain giving up, and so many, many more. Being caught in the pain of powerlessness is like being caught in a whirlpool, which pulls us deeper and deeper in the vortex—we go round and round and there seems no way to get out.

But there is a way, and again we're dealing with a paradox. We can lose the pain created by feelings of powerlessness by accepting that powerlessness as our reality. This is the bedrock of the Twelve Step program, and once we agree to it we can begin to use the Steps for our spiritual recovery.

When we admit to powerlessness we become humble, and humility can give us power. It relieves us of false pride, of grandiosity, and of the terrible tensions they can produce. We can be ourselves and not try to live up to the unrealistic expectations we may put on ourselves. It also relieves us of the pressure of sparring with others as we try to manage their perceptions of us. And when we accept humility we can redefine that expression we have hated—"at the mercy of"—into one that we understand means freedom. From humility we learn that we may feel powerless and still have a busy, active, stimulating, and involved life. We can have rich relationships with family and friends, contribute to our community, and have a fulfilling spiritual life. To be able to do all this while accepting our powerlessness means that we are beyond being threatened by life. To truly accept powerlessness and to go on with living is to find serenity.

But many of us have been taught that powerlessness is bad. It is such a negative that we may turn and run from it. Thus, we may never come to fully understand our powerlessness, explore its positive possibilities, or learn to be comfortable with its negatives. Our job while working the Fourth Step is to examine and understand the many facets of our powerlessness—without fear and without running away. The exercises that follow can help. The imagery exercise is designed to help us examine and become thoroughly familiar with that piece of us that is powerless, and the written exercise can help us see the place of powerlessness in everyday living.

Imagery Exercise to Find and Face Powerlessness

In your mind, let a symbol appear or a feeling arise that represents your powerlessness. The image could appear as a limp rag doll, or the sensation of being lost, or struggling in a swampy morass. You might see yourself as trussed up in a rope or naked and shivering with cold. Whatever the image is, look at it or sense it very carefully. Take time to really see it, to really feel it. Don't hurry this or be afraid—the symbol is in your imagination and it can't harm you.

Now ask your powerlessness to tell you exactly *what it is afraid of.* Listen to its answer. Don't interrupt, or argue, or try to make it feel better. Just listen.

Now ask your powerlessness *what it has to offer you.* Simply accept its answer quietly, no matter what it says, whether or not you approve, whether or not you agree, and no matter how strange it may seem.

Now ask your powerlessness *what it needs from you.* Again, just listen.

Now tell your powerlessness *what it has meant to you,* how it has helped you, how it has hurt.

As soon as you complete this conversation, write down on a separate sheet of paper what you have learned about your relationship with the part of yourself that is powerless. Repeat the exercise every day until the idea of powerlessness raises less tension and fewer negative feelings.

Written Exercise to Help Deal with Powerlessness

1. Describe a specific circumstance that makes you feel powerless. Explain exactly how you feel in the situation. List as many feelings as you can.

2. Describe, in detail, what you do to relieve the pain of powerlessness in that particular circumstance.

3. Think of your response in terms of the first three Steps of the Twelve Step program. Describe how your thinking and behavior might be different if you followed those Steps.

Repeat this exercise for as many circumstances as you can think of that lead you to feeling powerless.

Fear and Anxiety

When I have the inner strength to face my fear, I will not send it outward as hatred [or anger, or jealousy, or grief, or isolate myself because of it].

— *M.F., Touchstones**

Unlike much other emotional pain, fear is a natural human reaction to an unfamiliar or threatening situation. It is physiological, sending messages to our brain that lead us to fight or flee. We are threatened and choose to stand and battle the menace, or we decide that absence is the better part of good sense and leave. Sometimes when we are afraid we simply acknowledge our reaction as fear, but sometimes we are afraid and hide it under another emotion. I am afraid someone may hurt me in physical therapy, so I defend myself by lashing out in anger. I am afraid that my blindness will keep me from a job promotion, so I am jealous or blaming of my sighted competitor. I am afraid of how people react to my being in a wheelchair, so I isolate myself, cutting myself off from family and friends.

Franklin Delano Roosevelt, U.S. President from 1933 to 1945, gave us a key to spiritual growth, another way to serenity, when he said, "The only thing we have to fear is fear itself." Fear of our powerlessness can make us feel hopeless or despairing; without fear, we can look at life with anticipation, finding our own way. If we are not afraid of how others view our illness or disability, we will not blame them, or isolate ourselves—we can be enriched by life around us. If we are not afraid of the outcome of our condition, we can let go of grief—we can live each day to its fullest. And when we face our fears, accepting them for what they are and releasing them, our energy can be used to join with others instead of to fight or flee or to use as fuel for another

---

*Touchstones, Center City, Minn., Hazelden Educational Materials, 1986.

negative emotion. Our immune systems will not be impaired by the overproduction of stress hormones. We will be mentally healthier and more physically sound.

Because fear is a natural physiological response, it will always reappear. So we need to understand the fearful part of ourselves; we need to discover its strengths as well as its weaknesses. Then when fear comes we will know how to work with it so that it can be helpful and transitory instead of hurtful and controlling. Finding and facing our fear is central to our spiritual journey.

Imagery Exercise to Find and Face Fear or Anxiety

In your mind, let a symbol appear or a feeling arise that represents your fear or anxiety. Fear may appear as a dark, cloaked figure. Fear also often represents itself as a mass of blood or a writhing snake. You might see anxiety as a white field covered with squirming purple lines. Whatever the image is, look at it or sense it very carefully. Take time to really see it, to really feel it. Don't hurry this or be afraid—the symbol is in your imagination and can't harm you.

Now ask yourself exactly *what you are afraid of.* Listen to the answer.

Now ask your fear *what it has to offer you.* Simply accept its answer quietly, no matter what it says, whether or not you approve.

Now ask your fear *what it needs from you.* Again, just listen.

Now tell your fear *what it has meant to you,* how it has hurt you, how it has helped.

As soon as you complete this conversation, write down on a separate sheet of paper what you have learned about your relationship with the part of yourself that is fearful or anxiety-ridden.

Repeat the exercise every day until the idea of fear raises less tension and fewer negative feelings.

Written Exercise to Help Deal with Fear or Anxiety

1. Describe a specific circumstance that makes you feel fearful or anxious. Explain exactly how you feel in the situation. List as many feelings as you can.

2. Describe, in detail, what you do to relieve the pain of power-lessness in that particular circumstance.

3. Think of your response in terms of the first three Steps of the Twelve Step program. Describe how your thinking and behavior might be different if you followed those Steps.

Repeat this exercise for as many circumstances as you can think of that lead you to feeling fearful or anxious.

Isolation

I isolate myself because I'm ashamed, ashamed of how I look, ashamed of my weakness. When I'm around other people I'm so self-conscious—I can never forget that I'm different.

— *Sally, who has cerebral palsy*

Sally is ashamed of her disability. Like many chronically ill or disabled people, she isolates herself because of it. Shame is a paralyzing emotion. It says, "I am a mistake, the damage is be-yond repair, and the only thing is to reject myself and the world. I isolate myself because I don't want to have to explain myself to others, and when I'm out in public I feel like I always have to keep up a good front. The only place I don't have to do any explaining or keeping up is when I'm alone." This kind of isola-tion comes from being overly involved in others' reactions to our chronic illness or disability. We try to imagine what is happening in someone else's head and respond to it, instead of staying centered in our self.

Ellen, whose life is limited by debilitating arthritis, says, "I isolate myself because no one else can understand me." Some chronically ill or disabled people remain isolated in order to wallow in self-pity. Others act like martyrs, using their isolation as a tool of power to manipulate. And some angry people barri-cade themselves in isolation, taking the position of, "No one understands, so it's me against the world."

No matter what our reason, we may never gain spiritual health by holding on to isolation. Maybe it's possible for monks and mystics' spirits to grow in solitude, but they aren't ordinary people. For most of us, remaining apart denies our human need for sociability and intimacy and decreases our self-esteem. Self-esteem can't rise when we know we aren't making a contribution to our family or community.

It's hard to find positive effects from the pain of isolation, but there are possibilities. As long as isolation does not become a permanent emotional style, to live through it can give us a sense of security and competence. We know we can survive on our own. Also, it is possible to come out of a period of isolation with a strong sense of enjoyment of self. When we are content with ourselves, the time we spend apart from others changes from sad loneliness to joyful solitude. Finally, facing the misery of the isolated part of ourselves can lead to a loving self-nurturance that can raise our self-esteem and lead us to honest relationships with other people.

But all of the positive outcomes of isolation are dependent on one thing—coming out of it. Becoming content solely with our own company may cripple us with complacency, and nurturing our misery can lead us further into ourselves. We need to learn to leave our isolation behind.

To do this, we first need to understand what keeps us where we are: Is it shame? The impossibility of always keeping up a front? Feelings of being misunderstood? Or any of a myriad of other reasons? The reasons will be different, depending on our unique personalities and life circumstances. We can act "as if" (we enjoy getting together with other people). We can physically join the crowd, but until we understand our loneliness and isolation we will feel their consequences. The key is to examine our loneliness, to find the reasons that we isolate ourselves or feel isolated from others. Once we understand, meaningful action can follow.

Imagery Exercise to Find and Face Isolation

In your mind, let a symbol appear or a feeling arise that represents your isolation. Isolation can present itself as a desert, a huge snowfield, or a lonely, shrouded figure. Or you could see yourself locked in a clear plastic box. Whatever the image, look at it or sense it very carefully. Take time to really see it and feel it. Don't hurry this or be afraid—the symbol is in your imagination and can't harm you.

Now ask your isolation to tell you exactly *what it is afraid of.* Listen to its answer. Don't interrupt or argue. Just listen.

Now ask your isolation *what it has to offer you.* Simply accept its answer quietly, no matter what it says, whether or not you approve, whether or not you agree, and no matter how strange it may seem.

Now ask your isolation *what it needs from you.* Again, just listen.

Now tell your isolation *what it has meant to you,* how it has hurt you, how it has helped.

As soon as you complete this conversation, write down on a separate sheet of paper what you have learned about your relationship with the part of yourself that is isolated.

Repeat the exercise every day until the idea of isolation raises less tension and fewer negative feelings.

Written Exercise to Help Deal with Isolation

1. Describe a specific circumstance that makes you feel isolated. Explain exactly how you feel in the situation. List as many feelings as you can.

2. Describe, in detail, what you do to relieve the pain of isolation in that particular circumstance.

3. Think of your response in terms of the first three Steps of the Twelve Step program. Describe how your thinking and behavior might be different if you followed those Steps.

Anger and Rage

Powerlessness may be my basic fear, but it is this anger that's going to kill me.

— *Fred, who has had two heart attacks*

Fred's statement is true—for him, anger can be deadly. When anger is directed outward, toward other people, it can turn them away from us and we may become isolated. Then we typically use our leftover emotional energy to rationalize our behavior. But rationalization is a conscious process; our unconsciousness isn't fooled. It knows we have behaved badly and our self-esteem shrivels as our self-hatred grows. If we are the kind of personality that handles anger by turning it inward, it can cause depression, immobility, and apathy. This, too, results in isolation—and can block out any joy, contentment, satisfaction, or peace that we might otherwise feel.

On the other hand, anger focused at a specific, realistic target is a strong, useful human response to fear. If we can put aside unrealistic mental battles we can use the energy of anger to move us toward our goals.

Instead of projecting his anger outward by screaming at his physical therapist, or inward by refusing to cooperate, John, a young amputee, realistically focuses it on his situation and uses his angry energy to learn to walk. "I hate all this, I won't be a cripple. Just watch me walk now—and by God I'll go farther tomorrow."

Mary, who has breast cancer, feels at one moment like screaming at her husband and children and at the next like sitting in a closet and crying. Instead, she goes to the university medical library to learn all she can about her disease in order to take a more active role in her treatment.

Ella is 74 and has recently become wheelchair-bound by osteoporosis (a condition characterized by decrease in bone mass). She overcomes her inertia, turns off daytime television that is meaningless to her, and makes arrangements to join a senior day care program.

Each of these people has found an individual way to use the energy of anger. Each has learned not to displace it on to others or direct it inward, but to use it as fuel for emotional and spiritual growth.

A special relationship exists between anger and the Twelve Step program, particularly with the First and Second Steps. Most chronically ill or disabled people are angry. There are overt ragers, covert manipulators, and people who don't feel angry but are depressed—all from fighting the pain of powerlessness. As we take the First Step and stop fighting and stop trying to prove that we are in total control of our lives, we are led to accept our powerlessness and become humble. And humility and rage don't go together. As we take the Second Step, we gain hope that one day we will be healed from the scars of anger. Now, with Step Four, we prepare to do our part. We will find and face the ball of rage inside of us; we will search out its hiding places, so that ultimately we can use our anger constructively or let it go.

Imagery Exercise to Find and Face Anger and Rage

In your mind, let a symbol appear or a feeling arise that represents your anger or rage. Many people find some form of fire, the color red, or perhaps a huge wall that blocks off vision to symbolize anger and rage. Whatever the image is, look at it or sense it very carefully. Take time to really see it, to really feel it. Don't hurry this or be afraid—the symbol is in your imagination and can't harm you.

Now ask your anger and rage to tell you exactly *what it is afraid of.* Listen to its answer. Don't interrupt or argue. Just listen.

Now ask your anger and rage *what it has to offer you.* Simply accept its answer quietly, no matter what it says, whether or not you approve, whether or not you agree, no matter how strange it may seem.

Now ask your anger and rage *what it needs from you.* Again, just listen.

Now tell your anger and rage *what it has meant to you,* how it has hurt you, how it has helped.

As soon as you complete this conversation, write down on a separate sheet of paper what you have learned about your relationship with the part of yourself that is angry.

Repeat the exercise every day or so until the idea of anger and rage raises less tension and fewer negative feelings.

Written Exercise to Help Deal with Anger and Rage

1. Describe a specific circumstance that makes you feel anger and rage. Explain exactly how you feel in the situation. List as many feelings as you can.

2. Describe, in detail, what you do to relieve the pain of anger and rage in that particular circumstance.

3. Think of your response in terms of the first three Steps of the Twelve Step program. Describe how your thinking and behavior might be different if you followed those Steps.

Repeat this exercise for as many circumstances as you can think of that lead you to feeling anger and rage.

Ambiguity and Blame

Almost the worst thing about this whole situation is that I can't make sense out of it. Why did it happen? Why me? What's the point? Who do I blame?
    — Anne, 21, quadriplegic from a diving accident

Having a chronic illness or disability places us in an ambiguous situation, a situation where we can't figure out why things are as they are, what it all means, or what to do about it. As we struggle to make sense of our illness or disability, we may often turn to blame as a solution.

John, a man facing severe bypass surgery says, "My wife certainly could have done more to help. She wasn't very good at working out the doctor's diet—and, after all, she's the cook."

Elaine, just diagnosed with breast cancer and trying to understand what treatment options are open to her, asks, "Why? Why didn't I listen to what everyone said about quitting smoking? I was so strong-minded and dumb that I guess I deserve this."

For most people, being put in an ambiguous situation, particularly a negative one, leads to panic. We can't make sense out of it, so we are unbalanced and want an immediate and simple answer. The easiest way to find that answer and give meaning to the situation is to blame. Blame is almost reflex, whether we blame others or ourselves.

But blame is rarely useful. It almost always needs denial to maintain it; when we blame, denial controls our reactions and makes our decisions. And blaming leads to other hurtful consequences too. The heart patient, John, who blames his wife, makes her feel guilty; her anger matches his own, and the possibilities of their working out a cooperative post-surgical relationship are diminished. As a consequence, his future is further jeopardized. Elaine's self-hatred results in depression that impairs decision-making about her choices of treatment. It also impairs the function of her immune system, undermining whatever treatment she and her doctors finally decide on.

But there is an important positive effect from finding and facing the emotional pain of ambiguity and blame. We can learn to accept ambiguity as normal, face it calmly, study the situation from all sides, and ask for help from our Higher Power. Then we can rationally assess responsibility. Assessing responsibility means that we learn to recognize where responsibility lies without adding the emotional negatives of charging error or fault, without leaping into blame. As a result we can be released from denial, develop clarity in viewing our lives, and make responsible decisions. Also, we can become secure in our ability to face ambiguity, to face our future calmly, knowing that emotional pain and blame no longer control us.

Imagery Exercise to Find and Face Ambiguity and Blame

In your mind, let a symbol appear or a feeling arise that represents your ambiguity and blame. Perhaps you will see a fork in the trail ahead of you, or maybe you will get a sense of being in a dense fog. Or the symbol of an overbearing authority figure may come to you. Whatever the image is, look at it or sense it very carefully. Take time to really see it, to really feel it. Don't hurry this or be afraid—the symbol is in your imagination and can't harm you.

Now ask your ambiguity and blame to tell you exactly *what it is afraid of.* Listen to its answer. Don't interrupt or argue. Just listen.

Now ask your ambiguity and blame *what it has to offer you.* Simply accept its answer quietly, no matter what it says, whether or not you approve, whether or not you agree, no matter how strange it may seem.

Now ask your ambiguity and blame *what it needs from you.* Again, just listen.

Now tell your ambiguity and blame *what it has meant to you,* how it has hurt you, how it has helped.

As soon as you complete this conversation, write down on a separate sheet of paper what you have learned about your relationship with the part of yourself that feels ambiguous and blameful.

Repeat the exercise every day until the idea of ambiguity and blame raises less tension and fewer negative feelings.

Written Exercise to Help Deal with Ambiguity and Blame

1. Describe a specific circumstance that makes you feel ambiguous or wanting to blame others. Explain exactly how you feel in the situation. List as many feelings as you can.

2. Describe, in detail, what you do to relieve the pain of ambiguity and blame in that particular circumstance.

3. Think of your response in terms of the first three Steps of the Twelve Step program. Describe how your thinking and behavior might be different if you followed those Steps.

Repeat this exercise for as many circumstances as you can think of that lead you to feeling ambiguous or blameful.

Jealousy

It's funny, before the accident I used to like to read, and I even liked studying too. Now I couldn't care less about that stuff—all I think about is what I can't do. When I watch football on TV I really hate those guys because they can play and I never will again.

— Dave, paralyzed in a motorcycle accident

Dave, 19, is wheelchair-bound for life. He used to enjoy reading, thinking, and talking about ideas with his friends and parents. Now what he thinks about is how he hates the people involved in the freewheeling physical activities that are denied him. Jealousy and its partners—envy and resentment—form a painful, ugly trinity. This trio can separate us from others and deny us intimacy. There is simply no way to combine intimacy with envy or resentment or jealousy.

When we are jealous we focus on our weaknesses rather than on our strengths. We think about what we *don't* have instead of what we *do*. We think about what others have that we *don't*. We are apt to define things as negative rather than positive. We may look outside of ourselves for gratification rather than inside. And when we are jealous we often reject opportunities for positive and spiritually enhancing experiences.

Dave, the young paraplegic, refuses to meet with a teacher who wants to talk with him about tutoring a student who is failing Spanish. "It's a stupid idea—I help him raise his average so next year he can play varsity basketball when I can't."

Dave's jealousy has led him to shallow-mindedness and mean thinking.

Jealousy also can lead to obsession and increasingly narrows the limits of our thought.

Carol is in her mid-forties and had a mastectomy five years ago. She has been unable to decide whether or not to have her breast reconstructed. "I find myself noticing other women's breasts all the time. It's crazy but I can't help it. And when I see a woman with nice ones I hate her, I wish her bad things. That's crazy too. I'm not a mean or vindictive person but I'm so jealous I just feel nuts."

Carol is so completely tied up in her jealousy of other women that she can't realistically relate to her own situation. Her thinking whirls in narrow, obsessive circles.

The emotional pain of jealousy is hard to change because we often don't recognize it. We feel jealous, or resentful, or envious and try to get over it by arguing with ourselves, using reason to counteract unyielding emotion. This rarely works. If we peel back the grinding pain of jealousy, envy, or resentment and look beneath, we usually find the underlying pain is an encompassing sadness.

Finding our jealousy and facing the more basic pain beneath it gives us the chance to understand our deep sadness and insecurity. This understanding focuses our healing on basic hurts, rather than on the secondary pains of the ugly trinity. Then we can ask our Higher Power for help, our spirit can grow, and another step is taken toward serenity.

Imagery Exercise to Find and Face Jealousy

In your mind, let a symbol appear or a feeling arise that represents your jealousy. A common symbol for jealousy is the color green: sometimes it can be a field of color or sometimes an object. Whatever the image is, look at it or sense it very carefully. Take time to really see it, to really feel it.

Now, ask your jealousy to tell you exactly *what it is afraid of.* Listen to its answer. Don't interrupt or argue.

Now ask your jealousy *what it has to offer you.* Simply accept its answer quietly, no matter what it says, whether or not you approve.

Now ask your jealousy *what it needs from you.* Again, just listen.

Now tell your jealousy *what it has meant to you,* how it has hurt you, how it has helped.

As soon as you complete this conversation, write down on a separate sheet of paper what you have learned about your relationship with the part of yourself that is jealous.

Repeat the exercise every day until the idea of jealousy raises less tension and fewer negative feelings.

Written Exercise to Help Deal with Jealousy

1. Describe a specific circumstance that makes you feel jealous. Explain exactly how you feel in the situation. List as many feelings as you can.

2. Describe, in detail, what you do to relieve the pain of jealousy in that particular circumstance.

3. Think of your response in terms of the first three Steps of the Twelve Step program. Describe how your thinking and behavior might be different if you followed those Steps.

Repeat this exercise for as many circumstances as you can think of that lead you to feeling jealous.

Grief

When I was in it, there was no way I could have sorted it out.
You just don't realize that grief has taken over your life—and
you can't understand what's happened to you until it's over.
Getting back to normal is the only way to put it—during that
time I was absolutely not myself. Now I'd say I'm normal, but
I'm not the same person I was before it all happened.

— Jean, amputee

It's natural for chronically ill or disabled people to respond to the onset of illness or to a disabling accident with grief. The process of grieving, however, will be different for everyone, depending on the nature and severity of the condition and on the personality of the grieving person. Also, the pattern of a disease will make a difference. An illness with recurring remissions often keeps a person going through the same phases of grief, and a relentlessly debilitating disease means that there are ever-increasing losses to assimilate. A child disabled at birth may grieve periodically as she recognizes how the disability affects her life. Grief can be triggered on entering school, becoming a teenager, and moving into adulthood. As the disabled person matures, she begins to put together the emotional and psychological skills and strengths learned from the losses experienced during childhood and adolescence. Now, in adulthood, the changes may not come so quickly. Finally, there is time to resolve whatever grief she still may attach to her chronic illness or disability.

Grief is an emotional process that can take over our lives. It can control our relationships, our lifestyles, and our decisions. Researchers who study grief tell us that directly after any important loss, whether it's a divorce, retirement, death of a loved one, or the onset of a chronic illness or disability, we shouldn't make major decisions or plan radical changes in our lives. They say that to do so is foolish because our judgment is clouded and controlled by our grieving.

As difficult as it is to accept, grief is a protective mechanism for the mind. In the beginning it is a purely emotional reaction; intellect has little or no impact on it. In the first phase of grief, we use disbelief and denial to block out the seemingly unbearable fact of our illness or disablement — perhaps our mind needs to rest and gather strength to face the emotional storms to come.

Five years ago, Jean lost her hand in a factory accident. "When this first happened I kept telling myself to face reality. 'Your hand is gone. It's gone. You'll never have it back or be the same.' But I just couldn't feel anything; my mind was numb."

The second phase of grief acts as an emotional catharsis in which we bring feelings to the surface. These feelings can range from rage to disbelief. Jean explains what happened to her.

"When it hit, it hit with a fury. My emotions were wild, all over the map. They flipped around so fast and were so strong that I was sure I was going crazy."

But she wasn't crazy; she was just grieving. As we slowly move through this phase, our emotionally unbalanced system begins to right itself. Little by little, with many regressions, rationality and calm begin to reappear.

In the final phase of grief, we regain our psychological balance. We have a new definition of self, forged in the turmoil we have been through. We now become prepared to live life in terms of this new self-image. Jean relates her experience:

"I would never have asked for this to happen to me—and I will probably always wish it hadn't. But it has. What is, is. And in the process I've become a much stronger, probably a much better, person."

The resolution of grief is crucial for our spiritual health. As we move through the stages, our spirits evolve and real personal and emotional change can happen. Through grieving we can learn to admit our powerlessness and accept reality. We can let go of the past, ourselves as we were, our goals, our hopes and dreams. We begin to live honestly in today's situation, without denial, and we set new goals and dream new dreams appropriate to our current reality. We feel released, at peace with ourselves and with our world.

Imagery Exercise to Find and Face Grief

In your mind, let a symbol appear or a feeling arise that represents your grief. Grief can take the form of a deep pit or a rolling black cloud. Many people see a shrouded figure, standing alone. Whatever image you choose, look at it or sense it very carefully. Take time to really see it, to really feel it.

Now ask your grief to tell you exactly *what it is afraid of.* Listen to its answer. Don't interrupt or argue. Just listen.

Now ask your grief *what it has to offer you.* Simply accept its answer quietly, no matter what it says, whether or not you approve, no matter how strange it may seem.

Now ask your grief *what it needs from you.* Again, just listen.

Now tell your grief *what it has meant to you,* how it has hurt you, how it has helped.

As soon as you complete this dialogue, write down on a separate sheet of paper what you have learned about your relationship with that part of yourself that is grieving.

Repeat this exercise every day until the idea of grief raises less tension and fewer negative feelings.

Written Exercise to Help Deal with Grief

1. Describe a specific circumstance that makes you feel grief. Explain exactly how you feel in the situation. List as many feelings as you can.

2. Describe, in detail, what you do to relieve the pain of grief in that particular circumstance.

3. Think of your response in terms of the first three Steps of the Twelve Step program. Describe how your thinking and behavior might be different if you followed those Steps.

Repeat this exercise for as many circumstances as you can think of that lead you to feeling grief.

Exhaustion

One of the things that makes it so hard to deal with my arthritis is the sheer exhaustion that I feel. It's not depression; I'm just tired.
— *Ellen, whose life is limited by debilitating arthritis*

The exhaustion that comes with chronic illness or disability is based on both physical and emotional fatigue. This is not the debility of depression or the totally empty feeling of deep despair—but a realistic reaction to too much physical and emotional exertion. Physically, our disabilities can cause us to drain an excessive amount of energy from an already depleted body to carry out the activities in everyday life. It simply takes more energy for a man with multiple sclerosis to walk down the stairs than it does for his healthy wife. For a stroke patient, or a person with cerebral palsy, eating uses a concentration of energy that most of us just don't need as we maneuver knife and fork, moving food to our mouths.

Emotionally, our disabilities empty us too. We may be exhausted from experiencing or trying to control the emotional pains we attach to our condition. Sam, a man recently diagnosed with heart disease says, "I don't know which wears me out more: the anger I feel about all of this, or the energy it takes to keep my blood pressure down." We may be worn out by raging against our powerlessness, by repressing or fighting our fear, by maintaining our rationalization and denial as we blame, or by the ferocious mood swings of grief. And because of the isolation so many of us experience, we are kept from being energized by relationships with friends and loved ones.

But there are lessons to be learned from exhaustion. We can learn how to care for our bodies. We can learn how to strengthen them and invigorate them with exercise. We can learn how to pace ourselves, to find our own unique physical limits. We can learn how to fuel our bodies with good food, and learn which foods give energy and which ones deplete it. We can learn how to renew ourselves with rest, and know when to rest—what's too much or too little. We can learn how to be aware of our bodies and keep our physical condition in perspective. We gain the awareness of physical vulnerability earlier than most people do. To a chronically ill woman, aging doesn't come as a shock—she may not like what happens as she gets older, but she *knows* that her body is vulnerable to changes outside of her control. And we can learn to take real, conscious joy in simply feeling physically well. For a woman with arthritis, or a man with bladder cancer, a day free of pain is a joyful gift.

Exhaustion can teach us to care for our minds too. We become depleted from living with emotional pain, but as we learn to find, face, and release it, we develop mental techniques that will be lifelong guides for feeling free and alive. In giving up efforts to control our pain, in working the Twelve Steps, in asking for help from our Higher Power, we lose uncertainty, confusion, and exhaustion—and we find peace.

Imagery Exercise to Find and Face Exhaustion

In your mind, let a symbol appear or a feeling arise that represents your powerlessness. To many people, exhaustion appears as a sensation of nothingness—white or gray often are used as colors to symbolize exhaustion. Whatever the image is, look at it or sense it very carefully. Take time to really see it, to really feel it. Don't hurry this or be afraid—the symbol is in your imagination and can't harm you.

Now ask your exhaustion to tell you exactly *what it is afraid of*. Listen to its answer. Don't interrupt or argue. Just listen.

Now ask your exhaustion *what it has to offer you*. Simply accept its answer quietly, no matter what it says, whether or not you approve, no matter how strange it may seem.

Now ask your exhaustion *what it needs from you*. Again, just listen.

Now tell your exhaustion *what it has meant to you*, how it has hurt you, how it has helped.

As soon as you complete this dialogue, write down on a separate sheet of paper what you have learned about your relationship with the part of yourself that feels exhausted.

Repeat the exercise every day until the idea of exhaustion raises less tension and fewer negative feelings.

Written Exercise to Help Deal with Exhaustion

1. Describe a specific circumstance that makes you feel exhausted. Explain exactly how you feel in the situation. List as many feelings as you can.

2. Describe, in detail, what you do to relieve the pain of exhaustion in that particular circumstance.

3. Think of your response in terms of the first three Steps of the Twelve Step program. Describe how your thinking and behavior might be different if you followed those Steps.

Repeat this exercise for as many circumstances as you can think of that lead you to feeling exhausted.

CHAPTER EIGHT

CONSEQUENCES OF UNFACED PAIN

Living with the emotional pain we've been discussing has very specific psychological and behavioral consequences. We need to learn to recognize them before we can begin the process of changing to a more pain-free and rewarding life.

Denial—We pretend to ourselves that our condition doesn't exist, or doesn't affect us to the degree that it really does, or that it will go away if we ignore it. In other words, we deny our own reality.

Dishonesty—We evade the truth of our condition as we relate to others. We use half truths, distorted definitions, and constantly try to manage the impression we are making to maintain a charade. If our condition permits, some of us spend much time and effort in passing as healthy.

Intolerance—We become so rigid in our need to control our environment and so centered on our problems that we become intolerant, negative, and critical of others.

Self-pity—Our elaborate self-concern causes us to resent and reject others. We see ourselves as central to our entire social universe and feel self-pity when others aren't as consumed with our problems as we are.

False pride—False pride is pride based on the opinion of others. It develops when we reach for achievements and status that some people will judge as superior without regard to our own integrity, and when we hide our weaknesses and vulnerabilities. This is different from true pride that is based on our own opinion of ourselves and our comfort in showing vulnerability. We feel true pride when we are proud of an accomplishment because we have met our goals and have maintained our integrity. A stroke victim suffers false pride when she strives to walk because others will see her as "normal." She feels true pride when she is able to walk fifteen steps and congratulates herself for overcoming the tremendous physical odds against her.

These five characteristics come from excessive self-involvement; yet, in another way, they keep us alienated from ourselves. Our cycles of emotional pain separate us from our real self, the self we are trying to avoid, the self who is a normal person and who is chronically ill or disabled. Almost equally as devastating is that denial, dishonesty, intolerance, self-pity, and false pride keep us insulated from friendship and intimacy. Others may see our reality more clearly than we do; their vision is more objective. But in our pain and our need to control our environment we refuse to ask for, or accept, the assessments of friends and loved ones. Much as they care about us, they feel like outsiders— and we feel safer if we keep it that way.

A particularly harmful consequence of unfaced pain is the way we may use our emotional pain itself to control others. We may explode with anger, forcing others to "walk on eggshells" when they are with us. Or we use mood swings as tools of power.

The mother of a seventeen-year-old quadriplegic son says, "His mood controls the mood of the whole family. If he's up, so are we. When he's depressed we all feel awful and do anything we can to make him perk up."

Some of us become expert at using guilt to manipulate others. We get our way by making others sorry for us. Then, if they show their pity, we criticize them for making us feel "different."

Our friends and families are kept off balance; they aren't sure how to reach out to us. Some help by trying to read our minds and accepting our manipulative behavior; they become martyrs or codependents, people who spend their time trying to figure out what we want, without considering whether or not what we want might be hurtful or destructive to themselves. Some give up, relating to us only superficially or avoiding us. If we won't accept our reality as it truly is, if we continue to live within our cycles of pain, our friends and families are forced to do the same. Everyone loses—we are all deprived of intimacy, warmth, and spiritual growth.

But we don't have to live this way. Remember, our purpose in working the Fourth Step is to expose the harmful emotions and character traits that we have developed as a result of our chronic illness or disability—and to change them in a way that ensures our spiritual development. So far, we have made an inventory of emotional pains; in Steps Five, Six, and Seven we will discover a way to change them. As we prepare to give up the feelings that can destroy our spirits we need to briefly discuss the soul-enriching emotions that we can replace them with.

CHAPTER NINE

FILLING THE
VOID WITH POSITIVES

Hope: The Mainspring of Our Life Force

When we talk about spiritual fulfillment we speak of love, serenity, faith, joy, and often overlook hope. Yet hope is crucial. Without it our spirits could not evolve. The old saying, "Hope springs eternal in the human breast" is true. Hope is built into the psychological makeup of human beings; it's an integral part of us. We may take it for granted, but it's the mainspring of our life force. Hope is the energy that gets us up in the morning. It promotes enthusiasm, confidence, and joy. It lets us dream and set goals.

Another saying tells us, "As long as there's life, there's hope," and many seriously ill people use this belief to sustain their spirits when there isn't much else to cling to. It also works the other way: "As long as there's hope, there's life." Many doctors and their patients believe that medical miracles are simply hope given physical form.

Some people give up hope, make a clear decision, and die. They say, "I'm ready to go now," and they do. Doctors and nurses who work with terminally ill patients know it's not unusual for a patient to die if he or she gives up hope. Religions based on black magic work this way too. People are cursed, give up hope, turn their faces to the wall, and waste away. Psychologists cite case after case where clients lose hope and then lose their minds. And negative, self-fulfilling prophecies work because they, too, steal hope.

Hope fuels our life force, but hope needs to be applied realistically. This doesn't mean we shouldn't hope for the very best, but we can misuse hope when we use it to support denial. A man whose leukemia is in remission can hope that the remission will be a long one, but not use it to believe that he is cured. Rather, he must use the strength of hope to live his life as fully as he can, regardless of how long his disease is dormant. Hope may help his body heal, and it can make him spiritually strong.

Love: Nurturing Another's Spiritual Growth

Love is the will to extend one's self for the purpose of nurturing one's own or another's spiritual growth.

— *M. Scott Peck*
The Road Less Traveled

We don't usually think about love as an act of will. Perhaps we'd rather believe that it is happenstance, a feeling that descends on us from someplace or something—but that is not true. As any husband, wife, parent, lover, friend, caregiver, or person with a deep social conscience knows, love involves choice, intention, and action. To love is an act of one's will, and we love when we choose to exert ourselves in the cause of spiritual growth. So to will ourselves to love is to dedicate ourselves to the spirit.

Extending ourselves toward the spiritual growth of others can create the soul-fulfilling emotions of connection, intimacy, and true caring. It relieves our destructive self-centeredness and moves us out of ourselves into the human community. Sometimes our loving of others is perceived as supportive; we extend ourselves in ways that they like—as when we care for the pets of a hospitalized friend. Sometimes our loving is perceived in a different way—an alcoholic has trouble understanding his family's insistence of treatment as a loving act. But the bottom line is in the purpose. If the action is directed toward the nurturing of another's spiritual growth, it is love.

To extend ourselves toward our own spiritual growth is equally as important—and that is what the Twelve Step program does. This is a program of love designed to heal spiritual illness. When we choose the Twelve Steps as a guide, when we intend to work the Twelve Steps to rid ourselves of emotional pain, when we make the Twelve Steps our way of living, we are nurturing our spiritual growth. We are loving ourselves.

Joy: Remaining Open to Its Possibilities

Contentment, satisfaction, happiness: it's a wonderful moment when these good feelings surge up in us. Sometimes we plan for them—we set the stage, hoping to feel contented or satisfied, and we spend lots of time searching for whatever we call happiness. But joy is different. We can't create it. It's almost always unexpected. Pure joy is like a bursting light; it explodes and swells within us. And it's nearly always triggered by something spiritual. Joy is different from the exultation that comes from achievement or with the feeling of power. Exultation that comes from achievement can be soul-filling if the achievement is a loving one, if we know that it is useful to ourselves and others. But there is danger that it may encourage us toward achievement for its own sake. The exultation that comes with the winning of power is most often soul-destructive: it kills humility as it reinforces our desire to win, to be superior, to hold others beneath us.

True joy doesn't happen often. It comes with a flash of instant recognition of life and of love: the clear elegance of a flower, the green glory of a spring day, the beauty of a sleeping child, the soaring of a Beethoven violin concerto. For the fleeting moments it is with us, joy means total connection, connection with something greater than ourselves. In joy we connect with the universe—it is momentary, total spiritual fulfillment. We can't foresee joy, but if we remain open to its possibility, it will come.

Faith: The Miraculous Connection

Since the beginning of time people have created many different names and ideologies to try to explain the inexplicable force that operates our universe. But no matter what the force has been called, no matter what rituals and institutions have been developed around it, for all time and for all people one part of the process has been the same. That part of the process is the connection, the emotional relationship, between people and their God-force, the connection we call *faith*.

There is one entity, the human being, and another, the life force. These things can, and sometimes do, operate independently. If they are to get together, the current that runs between them must be faith; it is faith that activates the system.

Many people walk through life oblivious to the potential of the Power greater than themselves that surrounds them. They just don't have the faith to connect with it. On the other hand there are those whose lives are based on what Sören Kierkegaard, Danish philosopher and theologian, called the "leap of faith"— people who believe in a Power beyond themselves even when they cannot explain or touch it.

From the time we are children we hear that "faith can move mountains" or that "faith can make miracles." In real life the combination of our self, our faith, and our Higher Power may not move mountains but *can* create miracles. Some of us will experience major miracles, the kind Bernie Seigel talks about in *Love, Medicine, and Miracles*. But for most of us the miracles will be smaller. They will be unique, life-enriching experiences that will happen when we remain open to the possibilities in life and keep our faith turned on.

Serenity: Receiving Each Day's Joy

We may often think of serenity as calmness, peace, tranquility, a state of uninterrupted smoothness. To most of us, the monks and the Yogi meditators are examples of serene humans, and a gently flowing stream reminds us of serenity in nature. To be serene can be interpreted to mean to float through life, and serenity *can* be like this. We can have calm, tranquil times and they are wonderful. But the serenity we seek as a result of our spiritual evolution is not a passive state. On the contrary, it is a very active one. It means engaging with life, experiencing it fully, yet not being burdened by it.

Hans Selye, in *Stress Without Distress*, describes the differences between *stress* that promotes energy and that is a natural part of the human condition, and *dis-stress* that means being destroyed instead of energized by the pressures of life.

A fourth grade teacher goes energetically through her day with twenty-five students. Her energy can be serene energy moving without pressure and with love, or it can be dis-stressed energy fueled by impatience, frustration, and anger. The teacher experiences one set of circumstances but can respond serenely or with emotional turbulence.

To be serene is to live under stressful conditions without experiencing dis-stress.

Serenity is hard to come by. It requires that in our lives we surrender the outcome while we lovingly nurture and trust the process. We must stay present to the possibility of what each day offers and to receive its joy. For most of us, the way to accomplish this is by being deeply and consciously aware of the presence of our Higher Power that always stands with us.

Many other positive, constructive emotions can help fill the void left by our released pain. Our spirits are nurtured when we feel:

accepted	competent	enthusiastic	proud
appreciated	complete	fulfilled	relaxed
assured	confident	intimate	secure
calm	connected	loveable	satisfied
cheerful	curious	loving	wanted
comfortable	delighted	optimistic	wonder-full

We all know these feelings and others like them. They are natural emotions for everyone. Many of us with chronic illness or disability have had them blocked out by our pain, but now we need to encourage them—the more we feel them, the more they become our usual way of being, and the more our spirits will grow. What follows are two exercises that can help.

Written Exercise to Encourage Spirit-Enhancing Emotions

1. Describe a specific circumstance that makes you feel _____ (pick a feeling from ones described or listed in this chapter).

2. Describe circumstances or feelings that, for you, interfere with making you feel _____.

3. Think of your response as it relates to the first three Steps of the Twelve Step program and to the emotional pains discussed in the Fourth Step inventory. Describe how you might encourage your feeling of _____ if you use what you have learned.

Repeat this exercise for any of the spirit-enhancing emotions.

Imagery Exercise to Encourage Spirit-Enhancing Emotions

In your mind, let a symbol appear which represents _____ (pick a feeling from ones described or listed in this chapter). Look at it very carefully, take time to see and feel it. Don't hurry this; let the feeling come.

Now ask this feeling *what it has to offer you.* Simply accept its answer, no matter what it says.

Now ask this feeling *what it needs from you.*

Now tell this feeling *what it means to you, how it helps you.*

Finally, ask this feeling to return, again and again. Tell it you welcome it.

As soon as you complete the dialogue, write down on a separate sheet of paper what you have learned from this exercise about your relationship with this feeling.

Repeat this exercise for any of the spirit-enhancing emotions you would like to feel more often.

CHAPTER TEN

TAKING OUR STRUGGLE
TO THE OUTSIDE WORLD

Step Five: Admitted to the God of our understanding, to ourselves, and to another human being the exact nature of our wrongs.

In Step Four we made a searching and fearless inventory of ourselves. We examined the destructive and hurtful ways we have reacted to our illness or disability. We discussed the wrong thinking and wrong attitudes that have resulted in the emotional pain that keeps us from serenity.

Step Five is a turning point. It requires that we admit the exact nature of our "wrongs," first to ourselves and our Higher Power and then to another human being. As a result of the first four Steps, we have built the basis on which we can live a truly spiritual life, a life as our real selves. We have had an internal struggle, and now the Fifth Step asks that we take our struggle to the world outside of our own psyche. It makes the transition from thought to action, from intrapersonal to interpersonal, from isolation to connection.

We carried out the first Steps within our heads; now it is time to test our commitment to honesty and our willingness to face the consequences of our honesty. As we work Step Five, *The Little Red Book** promises us we will move from having a growth in spiritual *beliefs* to having a growth in spiritual *experience*.

Step Four may have been hard for us. It was hard to break through our denial and resistance to admit that the pains described were the pains we feel. It was hard to admit that we behave in ways destructive to ourselves and others. And it was hard to look at old feelings and memories that we have spent much time and energy hiding from ourselves.

On the other hand, there were many benefits to this hard work. There was relief in admitting the reality of our pains. We always knew they were there; our subconscious wasn't fooled by whatever pretenses our conscious mind concocted. Our hurt was no longer secret, a specter to be hidden and ashamed of. There was also relief in the hope that we could be pain-free. And Step Four gave us the opportunity to work closely with our Higher Power, nurturing ourselves as we found and faced our hated pain.

Step Five builds on Step Four and gives us the opportunity to complete the acknowledgment of our pain. We are asked to share the exact nature of our wrongs and the extent of our pain with ourselves, so we can accept our darker side and thus live whole. We also share our wrongs with our Higher Power, which increases our trust in that relationship. And we share those wrongs with another human being. This last part can be frightening— after all, we may have spent much of our time preventing others from seeing the feelings and emotions hidden inside us.

But when we carry out this Step we can have an experience that many of us didn't think was possible. As we open ourselves to another person's viewing, he or she will probably see our struggle, turmoil, nastiness, and aggression and not turn away. Instead of being repelled, the person will listen and understand.

---

*The Little Red Book. Center City, Minn.: Hazelden Educational Materials, 1970.

To most people this gives great release and relief—for some, it's a miracle.

Also, the Fifth Step gives us a firsthand experience in the power of humility. We may try so hard to feel powerful by keeping up a front, by controlling and managing the impression we make on others. Yet the humility required of us when we speak fully of our pain to another person can leave us truly powerful — not as in "having power over," which is superficial and externally based, but as in "being secure in self," which is internal and fundamental.

Finally, there is the value of public commitment. Telling another person of our intent is crucial to carrying out difficult tasks. Research by social psychologists shows that when we try to stop smoking, or go on a diet, or start an exercise program, if we tell other people about what we intend to do, we are much more apt to succeed. Going public benefits us in three ways. First, we receive a lot of support for our intended purpose; second, we find we can handle the response of those who disagree with us or who in other ways won't support us; and third, the guilt we would feel if we didn't carry through can help energize us into action. To be completely honest with another human being, to do a Fifth Step, is a start toward our public commitment to living an honest life.

Admitted to the God of our understanding, . . .

As we have taken the first four Steps we have become increasingly comfortable in contacting our Higher Power. Our trust in this all-loving and all-accepting Power makes the second part of Step Five seem a natural extension of talking with ourselves. One of the most important things we get when we fully admit our wrongs to our Higher Power is the experience of a non-threatening humility—we humbly share our pain and are received with caring.

Dan says, "Talking about it with my Higher Power seemed natural, easy. And I trusted that good would come of it—I'd get relief."

. . . to ourselves, . . .

This is perhaps the least difficult part of Step Five—we have been working at self-revelation from the beginning. We're used to it and getting pretty good at it, even though we may still deny having some problems in order to protect ourselves. By now most of us are fairly comfortable with getting to know parts of ourselves we haven't wanted to explore. And it's all in our own heads, so the risk is minimal.

Dan says, "After I really started to think about my anger, analyze it and see what it did to me, it wasn't so hard. Seeing it was there didn't make it any worse."

. . . and to another human being . . .

For most of us this is undoubtedly the most difficult requirement of Step Five. To allow another human being to see through our carefully managed presentation of ourselves to the turmoil within can seem impossible.

Jane, who has rheumatoid arthritis says, "I just didn't think I could do it. I'm sixty-three and felt like a scared five year old. No one has ever known how I feel about my arthritis, and I was proud of that fact. Now I had to talk about all the stuff I'd been hiding."

Jane did have to talk to another person; otherwise false pride would control her forever, and she would continue to avoid the responsibility of acknowledging her whole self, the negative as well as the positive. The experience of humility helped her spirit grow and increased her self-respect—and her honesty freed her from the tension of pretending.

When we choose a person to share our Fifth Step, we must choose with care. First and most important, we must feel safe and comfortable with the person. He or she must be objective and have the ability to keep what we say confidential. We should value that person's feedback because accepting that feedback is important in completing this Step. The person should be able to respond to us in terms of the beliefs and values of the Twelve Steps, and not just offer general advice. It is best to choose someone who is not a family member or close friend—with an insider, there often is too much history, too many preconceptions, and too many personal feelings involved. It is probably also best to choose a nondisabled person or at least a person who does not share the same physical problem—we need someone who can be completely objective. Remember, we have to admit the nature of our wrongs and the extent of our pain; we don't have to discuss changes or ask for help from our listener.

. . . *the exact nature of our wrongs.*

When we find and face our pain, the tendency is to label it as powerlessness, anger, fear, despair, or whatever. We identify it, but we try not to identify *with* it, try not to *feel* it. Labeling pain is a first step but only a first. It is one thing to say, "I am angry that I have diabetes." It is quite another to express that anger with all of the rageful emotion that our subconscious feels. If we do a Fifth Step with a listener and label and discuss our various feelings, it will help. But if we can express our feelings fully, detail them with examples, and show our deep vulnerability, it can help more. It is much harder, it may even deepen our own awareness of our pain, but ultimately this kind of revelation undercuts false pride, increases humility, and promotes complete healing.

Jane says, "I knew this was going to be one of the hardest things I'd ever done, but I was determined to do it right! I really opened up to her. I showed my feelings, didn't just talk about them. And once I started, it just got a life of its own and took off. I cried and laughed and beat on the arm of my chair. I was exhausted when it was over—empty and peaceful. My counselor was great. Didn't interfere with me at all. She just listened, and I knew that whatever I said was okay."

Jane was fortunate. She was able to decide, before she began, that she was going to carry the meeting through in the way she believed was in her best interest. She would do this even though it would be very difficult and contrary to all of her past behavior. Jane was able to put aside her self-consciousness, allow her vulnerability to show, and feel relief.

For others it may be a little more complicated. When they break through their denial to the exact nature and extent of their pain they find an overwhelming wall of shame—shame about the pain and about the chronic illness or disability that causes it. That happened to Meg, who has been blind since a freak accident.

"When I was talking, I was washed with feeling—but not the feeling I was talking about. Instead I was overwhelmed with shame."

It's shame that supports denial, and talking with another person about the exact nature and extent of her wrongs broke Meg's denial. It exposed her shame, and allowed her to work on that shame with a caring, accepting person.

Step Five shows us the way out of isolation and loneliness. It teaches us that we can be our whole selves without being rejected or abandoned. It lets us see that we have the strength to face the pain within ourselves and to show it to others. It lets us see that humility can bring us into the human community.

After completing a Fifth Step we may feel different, relieved, exalted, or we may feel that it is just another necessary Step in a lifelong process. It doesn't matter. The only important thing is carrying it out to the very best of our abilities.

We must not expect miracles—insight and one cathartic experience aren't enough for real long-term change. We may lapse again and again. We may become servants to our pain, which we try to deny and hide. But each time we recover, each time we recommit to honesty, each time we turn to our Higher Power for support, we make it easier for ourselves in the future. Learning to live with humility and honesty may be more difficult than learning many other things, but the technique is the same: practice, practice, and more practice.

After we do a Fifth Step we find that we have two supports — our Higher Power and the memory of our Fifth Step experience. We can carry these supports with us as we slowly begin to live honest and humble lives, free of pridefulness, deceit, and grandiosity. In our new regime of honest living we will need these supports. We will need them because while most people will accept and value our new beliefs and behaviors, some people, perhaps even some we love, may be uncomfortable with our change and reject us.

Many people repeat their Fifth Step from time to time. It's a good idea for two reasons. First, it reinforces a belief in our capability to be honest with ourselves, our Higher Power, and other people. Second, in repeating the experience we can always deepen it; we can get more and more away from simple identification of our pain and into closer identification with it. The more we know about it, the more we feel it, the more of it we will be able to it.

Step Five: Written Exercise

1. List the emotions you felt when you admitted the exact nature and extent of your pain to: (a) yourself; (b) your Higher Power; and (c) another person. Make each of these lists as detailed as possible.

2. How was the feedback you received when you talked about your pain with another person helpful to you?

3. Were there ways in which you felt hurt by the feedback? If so, list them.

4. List the things you felt most uncomfortable about sharing with your Fifth Step person.

5. Were there things you felt you couldn't talk about? If so, what were they?

6. How do you feel about having completed the Fifth Step? How has it benefitted you?

7. How do you feel about repeating this Step in the future?

Step Five: Imagery Exercise

Close your eyes and imagine yourself in a safe place. Comfortable and relaxed. You are aware that you are going to do something difficult and that it will come out well. Enjoy the feeling.

Now start thinking of all the pains you experience with your chronic illness or disability. Think of each of them and how they hurt you. Allow yourself to experience this.

Now ask your Higher Power to join you. Explain what you are feeling and why.

Now ask the person you have chosen to do your Fifth Step with to join you and your Higher Power. If you feel frightened, ask your Higher Power for comfort.

Now imagine yourself talking about the exact nature and extent of your emotional pain. Imagine being as vulnerable as you are able. Watch yourself carefully, and notice how your Higher Power supports you. Take your time; don't rush this.

Now when you have said everything you want to, thank your Fifth Step person and your Higher Power for being available to you.

Now open your eyes and return to your day.

Giving Up Our Pain

Step Six: *Were entirely ready to have the God of our understanding remove all of our defects of character.*

The traditional words of A.A.'s Sixth and Seventh Steps may seem harsh. We don't like to feel as though we have "defects of character" or "shortcomings." But what these words really mean is that we are human—that we have attitudes and behaviors that lead us to live with emotional pain. Our job is to work with the Steps so that our "defects," "shortcomings," and self-destructive attitudes and behavior will be replaced by strength, integrity, and faith.

Step Six asks again for deep introspection. We get a chance to look at the effect unconscious motivation has on our lives. First, it questions our readiness to change. Are we entirely, absolutely, ready to give up the way we have learned to be, the way we are? Are we ready to live without the emotional pain attached to our chronic illness or disability? Are we ready to give up the behaviors that go with that pain? Second, this Step questions our commitment to trusting and having faith in our Higher Power. Do we believe that our Higher Power cares enough, or is strong enough, to help us? If we are ready to give up our pain and our dysfunctional behaviors, and if we do believe in our relationship with our Higher Power, Step Six assures us of spiritual growth.

Were entirely ready . . .

When asked, "Are we ready to live without emotional pain and the destructive behavior that goes with it?" our immediate response is, "Of course, who would want to continue this way?" And the hard answer to that is, "We would."

Early in our chronic illness or disability we may have taken on emotional pain and destructive behaviors as the best response to the situation at that time; they were the least threatening of all possible reactions. This seems hard to believe, but remember, for the most part we don't learn and maintain feelings and actions that we don't want or that don't help us survive. They may be poor choices. But to us they may seem like the least of the evils. We make a conscious decision to define, feel, and behave in a certain way, and those reactions can become ingrained and habitual. We may become comfortable with our pain—it is a known quantity, and we are practiced in handling it. We may choose to stay with the predictability of our current way of being.

In many ways our pain may have protected and "helped" us. Shock and denial protect us from the mind-shattering pain of initial discovery or diagnosis of our chronic illness or disability. Feelings of powerlessness are realistic responses to a situation beyond our control. Fear, anxiety, depression, and grief all can act as tools of power. We may gain a sense of control as we use them to manipulate the feelings and behavior of other people. Grief and powerlessness can get us support. Anger, rage, blaming, and isolation may keep others at a distance. Pain can keep our attention on ourselves; this may feel safer than having to take risks with others. And pain can protect us from having to accept ourselves and get on with life and personal growth. Our pains "help" us to feel as though we are in some way controlling and managing our lives. They are predictable; we know how they work.

In working the Sixth Step, keep in mind we are dealing with our irrational, subconscious mind, rather than our rational consciousness. Our subconscious mind tries to maintain the status quo—fighting hard against any decision our conscious mind makes toward change. This is understandable. We face several powerful threats if we choose to accept our whole selves and begin to live without pain.

First, there is the issue of predictability and security mentioned earlier. We may not like how we feel and act, but we are familiar with it—there are no surprises. Second, and closely related, is our fear of the unknown and of taking risks. Third, there is the question of the void. If we let go of our present emotions, what will we put in their place? How do we do those other things? For most depressed people the idea of being outgoing and active is so frightening that they feel physically sick when they think about it. Those filled with rage and anger often say, "If I imagine that it [the anger] is gone, there's this empty place in me." Or, "If I'm not angry, then what's going to push me?"

Finally (and this is our subconscious mind's trump card for keeping us from change), there is fear of facing what our pain is trying to hide. We are who we are: chronically ill or disabled people. This is our life, our only life; we are going to live it within constraints that most people don't experience and can't understand. So—given these threats, no matter how much we think we want to rid ourselves of pain and negative behavior, things will not change until our subconscious mind is ready to have them change.

Spiritual growth, the very heart of the Twelve Step program, takes place through our subconsciousness. Our conscious mind has done what it can: it has lectured us, threatened us, bargained with us, pleaded with us to let go of our pain and change our ways—and it hasn't worked. Now we need to let the Twelve Steps take over. We need to allow our Higher Power to work within our subconscious mind, to nurture us, to hear us, to melt away the threat. With the Sixth Step we recommit ourselves to the care of a Power greater than ourselves. Our faith in this Power and our trust that it can remove our pain and therefore change our lives is our foundation of strength and hope.

. . . *to have the God of our understanding remove all of our defects of character.*

Step Six doesn't require that we take charge of removing our self-destructive behaviors and our pain. It centers on the fact that we can't do it by ourselves. In A.A. it's often said, "You alone can do it, but you can't do it alone." We don't need to be active; all we must be is ready. We simply allow ourselves a state of mind, a state of being, that is willing to let go. We must be willing to surrender our pain to our Higher Power, to be willing to finally live without it. Our ability to do this is a measure of our humility. As in Step Three, we must give over our will and our ego, to truly place them in the care of our Higher Power. It is the will of this Power that can remove our pain, not the will of our conscious mind.

Some people come easily to the point where they feel entirely ready to have their pain removed; some think they are ready but find their will still in control and refusing to let go. Most of us move very slowly in this Step. To help, some of us use The Serenity Prayer.

> God grant me the serenity
> To accept the things I cannot change,
> The courage to change the things I can,
> And the wisdom to know the difference.

Some of us create our own version of this traditional prayer. Some have other affirmations, mantras, or meditations that they find meaningful and helpful. Slowly and with much effort we move toward the place where we can believe in life without our pain. Slowly we deepen the humility that will make that life possible. Slowly we move on toward the Seventh Step.

Step Seven: Humbly asked God to remove our shortcomings.

To successfully work the Seventh Step we must have self-respect, we must be humble, and we must exercise faith. These three elements come together into a process that works to remove emotional pain. To honestly ask our Higher Power to help us, we must respect ourselves enough to believe that we deserve to live without pain—we must believe in our personal value and integrity. We have indicated this self-respect by deciding to practice the Twelve Steps and by dedicating ourselves to personal growth. As we do this, we say, "I'm looking for a better way; I'm worth struggling for." To accept ourselves and our place, without denial or grandiosity, is to be humble. We must be humble if we are to sincerely ask for help and to sincerely receive it. Exercising faith gives us the energy that makes the process work. We may have self-respect and be humble, but without the energy of faith we cannot have a relationship with a Higher Power, and our pain cannot be removed.

Humbly asked God . . .

With Step Seven we don't request, plead, insist, or bargain; we "humbly ask" our Higher Power to remove our pain. To be humble is the requirement. Humility is a natural consequence of the

Twelve Step program, and only through humility can we live it. Step One asks us to understand humility by accepting our powerlessness; Step Two requires that we acknowledge a Power outside of and greater than ourselves. The Third Step deepens our humility by suggesting that we turn over our life and will to this Power in the belief that it, better than we, can lead us to spiritual growth and fulfillment. The Fourth and Fifth Steps increase both our humility and self-respect as we identify, accept, and acknowledge to another person the extent of our shortcomings. Finally, in Steps Six and Seven our humility allows us to ask for the active intervention of our Higher Power.

. . . *to remove our shortcomings.*

We need to put ourselves in a frame of mind in which our shortcomings can be removed. We have to be willing to let go of our self-destructive feelings and be available to our Higher Power. So—how do we do this?

Delores, who is being treated for a melanoma (a malignant tumor) on her back says, "All I say is help, help. I don't ask anything."

Cathy has just had an ileostomy (a permanent removal of her lower bowel) to relieve her life-threatening colitis. She doesn't ask for help, just admits her pain, over and over: "I am so angry, I am so angry."

Although talking with our Higher Power is a very individual thing, here are suggestions to make this dialogue more effective: Especially important is remembering the kind of request that begins, "I want to _____" (be less angry, feel more secure) doesn't work. We are asking our Higher Power to support our will, and the whole point of Step Seven is to acknowledge that our will hasn't worked, that we need to look to the will of a Power greater than ourselves to relieve us.

Because our pains and behaviors are so habitual, it's often hard to recognize them when they occur. Some people find it helpful to imagine a separate part of themselves that stands outside to observe. The job of this observer is not to be judgmental or critical but to be objective. When the observer notices a negative feeling or a behavior that represents this feeling, it can call for help from a Higher Power.

Another thing that helps is to try new behaviors, to ask for ways to break out of old patterns.

Rhoda says her husband gets impatient when he gets tied into her dialysis routine. "Sometimes he has to rearrange business meetings to take me to an appointment when, for some reason, I can't drive myself or there's some other kind of problem. I used to always feel guilty, hurt, and angry, but I wouldn't say anything. I would just go out of my way to try to make it up to him.

"Then, one day, when this process started and I got the old feelings, I stopped and asked my Higher Power to tell me how this could change. Lo and behold, I got the idea to make an arrangement with a neighbor, Rosalie. If I could count on her to take me to dialysis when I couldn't get there by myself, she could count on me for emergency baby-sitting in return. Then I told my husband about how I felt and what I'd worked out with Rosalie. He felt guilty at first, but we talked about that, too, so now it's a lot better. I don't know why I didn't think of this sooner—my Higher Power has great ideas, but I was so busy feeling miserable I couldn't hear them."

In the course of living with our disability or illness, we have learned patterns of behavior that have become deeply ingrained habits. Even though many of them are unhealthy and may increase our pain, they are behaviors we know and it will take much hard and committed work for us to allow our Higher Power to remove them. We can go slowly, remembering the strength of "one day at a time." Some of our steps will be baby steps; we will lose a little fear in one situation, and be relieved of a little anger in another. We can acknowledge the change, be grateful for it, and look forward to more. Some of us may experience giant steps. We may wake up on the other side of depression or find ourselves going to bed at night with surplus energy. We may never lose all of our negative feelings, but we can learn to use the negative feelings we have left in positive ways. Instead of feelings of isolation filling us with the pain of loneliness, we can use them to indicate a need to separate from others and rest. Our powerlessness can increase our awareness of our relationship with our Higher Power. We can use anger as constructive energy, rather than in ways that hurt ourselves or others. And we can use fear as an impetus to search for knowledge about whatever it is we're afraid of.

For the Seventh Step to work it doesn't matter how we perceive our Higher Power; all that's necessary is that we have self-respect, are humble, and have faith that whatever we see as that Power can help us.

Meg's God is a traditional one. She prays: "Please see my pain and help me to understand Your Will for me. My life is in Your hands."

Dan's Higher Power is the Twelve Step program. He asks: "Help me live by the principles of the program. Help me let go of my pain and find a better way."

Jane, whose Higher Power is a White Light inside herself, never really asks for help. "I just decided to concentrate on living the program as I understood it. My fears about my future have evaporated—today seems more important than tomorrow. And rarely, rarely do I get angry or discouraged anymore. There's no reason to. I am who I am and that's good."

Step Six and Seven: Written Exercise

1. As you begin to work Step Six, ask yourself how ready on a scale of one to ten you are to have your Higher Power remove your shortcomings.

2. Of the eight major emotional pains described in Step Four's inventory, which play the biggest role in your life?

3. Which destructive feelings have been most useful to you? Describe how.

4. Which of them will be most difficult to let go? Why?

5. Which will be easiest to release?

6. Which of them do you think have the potential of acting as positives instead of negatives? How will this work for you?

7. How can your subconscious mind control your emotional pain?

8. Why does humility play such an important role in working Steps Six and Seven?

9. What is your most effective way of communicating with your Higher Power?

Steps Six and Seven: Imagery Exercise

Imagine yourself in a safe place. You are relaxed and comfortable. Your Higher Power is with you.

Now imagine a painful feeling. Allow an image that represents that feeling to come into your mind. Your Higher Power is quietly with you as you allow this image to appear. Take time. Let your subconscious mind give you whatever it will. When you can see or sense the presence of your negative feeling, take it in your hands. Take time to experience how it feels to hold it.

Now allow your Higher Power to take it from you. Remain completely willing to let go. As it is taken from you, notice what happens to the image. Notice also how it feels to give away your pain. Stay with that feeling—if you are uncomfortable, ask your Higher Power for support; if you are relieved, give thanks.

Now open your eyes. Repeat this exercise as often as you wish. Either repeat it with the same pain or use it for others.

CHAPTER ELEVEN

MAKING AMENDS

Step Eight: Made a list of all persons we had harmed, and became willing to make amends to them all.

"Impossible!" . . . "No way!" . . . "How would I dare!" These are all common responses to what the Eighth Step asks of us. "There are just too many people. My friends, my family, doctors, nurses, lab techs, and receptionists—there's no end to it." And seemingly there is no end. Once we truly accept how we have behaved, many of us are overwhelmed by the enormity of what working Step Eight would mean.

Also, we are frightened by the new pain we may face. "Just the thought of looking at all that makes me so guilty, I can hardly stand it. Can't I just forget the past and get on with what I am doing with myself now?" The answer is, "No." In the first place, we can't forget the past; we can only gear up our denial to suppress it. The best we can do is use our emotional energy to push it into our subconscious where it will continue to influence us. This is the way we have done things in the past, and we know that hasn't worked. It's denial, it's dishonesty, and it's self-destructive.

When we get past our immediate rejection of the idea of making amends, we can slow down and think about it. The Twelve

Steps have given us the tools to atone for our past. We know what it means to be honest, we have faith that our Higher Power is with us and will care for us, we have an increased sense of self-respect, and we have the experience of the Fifth Step to carry with us. All we need to do is to allow ourselves to spend whatever time we need nurturing ourselves, communicating with our Higher Power, and just getting used to the idea.

When we are faced with an enormous problem, it always helps to break it down into smaller pieces. First we'll look at our feelings about what we have to do and then clarify what making amends actually means.

Most of us are afraid of the feelings we will have if we face the people we have harmed and acknowledge how we have harmed them. We may be afraid we will look foolish or may be afraid of guilt, regret, remorse, or shame. Guilt and regret are healthy responses in this situation. Guilt, which comes when our behavior conflicts with our personal values, is certainly appropriate. And regret, which means to look back on an event with sorrow or to be distressed because of it, makes good sense too. But remorse (self-accusatory regret) and shame (the viewing of ourselves as worthless) are unhealthy responses. We need to carefully search our reaction and decide which of these emotions we are feeling. Then we need to turn to our Higher Power to help us deal with false pride, remorse, and shame.

When we think of making amends, most of us think of apologizing—and that's wrong. Amends are not apologies. Apologies are saying we're sorry, amends are changing our behavior. Many times in our anger we lash out at a friend or loved one. Then we apologize. Then we become angry and lash out again. Then we apologize. And on and on. Nothing changes. Amends may include an apology but are also much more. When we make an amend, we acknowledge what we have done, accept full responsibility for it, make a commitment to change our behavior, and try never to repeat the harmful action. This is a true amend. It's very hard, but it's not impossible. And it's essential for spiritual wellness.

After working the first seven Steps, we have come to realize that it's important for us to let go of the past and to put our emotional energy into living in the present. Amends are important because we cannot build a good present when our hurtful past lies hidden in our subconscious. It eats up our energy and keeps us bound to old feelings that may interfere every day of our lives. The only way to break this tie is to let go of our denial about the past. We can admit that in our pain we have hurt ourselves and others. We can make our amends. Then we can learn to be honest in the present, to respect ourselves, and to treat others with honesty and respect as well. The Eighth Step prepares the way for that to happen.

Made a list of all persons we had harmed, . . .

This list starts with our own name. It's imperative that we make amends to ourselves first; otherwise we can't sincerely or effectively make amends to others. It's like love and respect—we have to give it to ourselves before we can pass it on.

Our commitment to living by the Twelve Step program is the foundation for making amends to ourselves. We are committed to changing our thoughts, beliefs, and our behavior. Until now, we may have abused ourselves. We may have accumulated hours, days, months, perhaps years of abusing our minds with the stress of negative emotions. We may have exchanged days and nights of our lives for pain—pain we cannot manage. We may have also abused our relationsips with others. So we have lost lots of time, and we have lost friends, loved ones, and intimacy.

As we work the program and make amends to ourselves we can take time to grieve our losses. We can use our Higher Power to help us deal with the emotions involved in our grieving.

When we have made amends to ourselves, we can begin the process of making amends to others. On our list we put anyone and everyone we can think of who we have harmed. It can include spouses, children, parents, lovers, friends, colleagues, and acquaintances. Sometimes we may have been deliberately hurtful. Sometimes we were blind to the injury we may have caused others as we focused all of our thoughts on ourselves. We may have caused harm by lashing out in anger, resentment, or jealousy. Or we may have harmed silently, keeping our negative feelings inside where they can poison relationships.

We can hurt others when we use powerlessness to make them feel guilty and manipulate them. We may use our rage as an emotional battering ram. In our isolation we may be unaware of the needs of loved ones or how our rejection hurts our friends. Our pain, denial, and dishonesty can cut us off from intimacy with others and cuts others off from the potential of our affection and caring. Absolutely no one wins.

Many, many people may be on our amends list, and as we write it we are apt to forget that it took a long time to get here. We may not be able to make all our amends immediately. And that's all right. How long this takes is not important; it simply needs to be done and we need to be willing to begin the process.

. . . and became willing to make amends to them all.

Making amends is another form of public commitment: when we begin, the word spreads, and our relationships change with many people.

We must be willing to do four things. First, we must fully accept our part in any situation where something we have done, or not done, has injured someone else. No matter how justified we may have felt at the time, we must acknowledge our harmful act. Second, we must be willing to forgive both ourselves and others. Often those we harm, harm us in return—or maybe it was their harming us that caused us to retaliate. Nevertheless, we must forgive them, and accept our part in the interaction. Third, we must be willing to take the consequences of our amends with humility and search for ways of restitution. Finally, we must carry all of this out to the very best of our abilities and then be willing to let go of it forever—to turn it over to our Higher Power.

Growing Stronger

Step Nine: Made direct amends to such people wherever possible, except when to do so would injure them or others.

Beginning to take the Ninth Step is like standing on the threshold of a new life. We are learning to live with humility and honesty in the present, but if this new life is to have real integrity we must put our past life in order. We want to build our house on firm ground, not quicksand. Step Eight has led us to this point: we know what we need to do; now we have to *do* it. To ourselves, we have acknowledged the ways in which we have hurt others. Now we must acknowledge that hurt to each of our victims.

Not only does working the Ninth Step help us to resolve our past, it also strengthens the special traits that help our spirits grow. It takes courage to stand face to face with someone we have truly harmed and say, "I know that I hurt you, I am responsible for doing it, I deeply regret it, and I pledge to you that I won't ever do it again." It takes insight, thoughtfulness, and wisdom to choose the amend that will be most beneficial to each individual we have harmed. It takes patience, reflection, and planning to find the most appropriate time and method to carry out our amends. It takes a deep understanding of our need to resolve the past in order to free ourselves for the future. Finally, it takes vigilance to protect ourselves against the denial that could cause us to avoid a particular amend.

Making amends is an ongoing process of resolving our emotional conflicts, not something we can do quickly and get it over with. Carrying them out in a thoughtful, thorough way becomes a part of life as we work the Twelve Steps. It continually deepens our humility. As our spirituality grows, we may recognize more situations in which our pain has hurt others and know that the only way to erase that hurt for both the other person and ourselves is to make an amend.

Carrying out Step Nine can bring great benefits. Each time we do an amend we lose guilt and resentment and gain self-respect, courage, confidence, and self-esteem. This can happen no matter how the other person responds. When the person accepts our amend and supports our efforts, we grow. When it goes badly, when the other person is angry, disrespectful, and lashes out at us, we still know that we have done all in our power to take responsibility for our actions, so we grow from that too. To endear ourselves to the people we have harmed is not the object; the object is to live one day at a time with self-respect and integrity.

Made direct amends to such people wherever possible, . . .

Making a direct amend means to take candid, straightforward action. What form that direct action takes will depend on the availability of the person involved. If he or she lives nearby or can be easily reached, we should meet that person face to face. This is the most intimate, and therefore probably most effective way of presenting an amend. It is appropriate to telephone first, explaining that we would like a meeting. We don't have to give any special reason; it's better not to get bogged down in an explanation at this point.

Most people find it harder to go to enemies than to friends or loved ones, but for some, the closer the relationship with the harmed person, the more difficult the amend. Some of us like to make our most difficult amends first, to get them over with; some start out with less threatening amends to "practice on the easier ones" or "work up to the toughies." If we reflect on this, ask for the advice of our Higher Power and quietly wait for a response, we will know who to contact first.

In a few cases, the person we have harmed may be unaware of what we have done and not know we suffer guilt and regret because of it. It's very easy to avoid these amends. *What difference does it make?* we may think to ourselves. *She doesn't know, so why should I upset things?* The fact that she may not be aware of what we have done is irrelevant for Step Nine; it's our awareness of wrongdoing that matters. It's our subconscious that must continue to carry the pain until we make the amend. When we have the courage to approach our unaware victims, we show the depth of our commitment to the Twelve Steps and our intent to live an honest and humble life. The visit may be awkward and have consequences we don't like, but to avoid it is to allow old patterns of denial and rationalization to take over. To carry it through enriches our spirit.

We will probably need to make amends with some people it is impossible to meet face to face. They may live too far away or for some other reason be unavailable. These amends can be made by telephone or we can write letters. Phoning is the more direct way, because we have to deal with the other person's immediate response. It's often useful to follow up our call with a letter. Avoiding the telephone and making the amend by mail alone is attractive because it's easier, less threatening. But it is a one-sided communication, the least effective method, and it side-steps our responsibility.

It's just as important to make amends to people who we can't contact at all because of death or due to losing touch with them. There are several ways to do this. We can have conversations with them, either in our imagination, or, more effectively, by pretending we are with them. We visualize them sitting with us and make our amends out loud to them. This is our way of putting the relationship to rest and releasing ourselves at the same time. Another method is to write a long, detailed letter to the person, even though it will never be mailed. Finally, we can make our amend to someone who has died or disappeared by searching out and assisting a relative or other individual important to the person we harmed. We can explain our motivation, or we don't have to, whichever seems appropriate.

Making Your First Amends

Certain guidelines can help when we plan to make amends.

1. Plan. Be sure of what you want to say. Be thorough in your preparation. Spend as much time as you need with your Higher

Power, asking advice and listening to the response. Each amend will be different, based on the situation, so plan carefully each time.

2. Don't go into it with expectations about how the other person will respond. Simply be respectful and understand that you must accept whatever happens. You don't have control over the outcome, only over your part in the process.

3. Ask permission first and be willing to accept the other's response. Some victims may not accept your amend and that's their right. We must not gain our peace of mind by being disrespectful.

4. Be careful to take the responsibility for what happened on your shoulders. Speak only of your part in the hurtful situation; don't comment on behavior of the other. If you have any remaining resentment or anger, the amend won't work.

5. Keep it simple.

6. Whatever the other's response, remain humble, without anger or resentment.

7. Be willing to forgive yourself and the other person, and when the amend has been made release your pain to your Higher Power.

Jane, suffering from rheumatoid arthritis, and Dan, with heart disease, both had a great deal of anxiety as they began to work Step Nine. Jane chose to approach a friend, while Dan made his first amend to one of his original doctors, who had died.

Jane: *"I met with her and told her I knew how my rejection of her offers of help and friendship had hurt her. I was very explicit about the specific pain that I was suffering that made me act the way I did. I asked for her forgiveness, but told her that whether or not she could forgive me, I wanted her to know how deeply I regretted that I had locked her out of my life. She didn't exactly fall into my arms, but we are working out a new relationship. Her trust is growing. We're still friends."*

Dan: "*I wanted to make an amend to my first doctor. He tried hard to help me, but I was so mad at that point and I took most of it out on him. When he died, I felt guilty but put it out of my mind. So for the Ninth Step I wrote him a letter. I told him how angry I was at that time, how I knew that I'd been awful to him, and that I really felt sorry about it now. I know how hard he tried to help me; he was a good person and a good doctor. And I told him how I was doing great now. I actually cried when I wrote it. Then I wrote a letter to his wife and told her how important her husband had been to me, that he had been a fine man. It's okay to think about him now; I feel much better.*"

. . . except when to do so would injure them or others.

There is an exception to making direct amends. If we think we might harm someone by making a full amend to them, or that our disclosures might hurt a third person, we need to be very careful about how we proceed. First, we must be sure that we are not rationalizing our avoidance, that our concern is genuine. Prayer, meditation, and consultation with an objective outsider helps. If we decide that a partial amend is necessary to avoid giving the other person more pain, it's appropriate to set limits on what we say. This kind of amend will protect the victim, and give us full benefit, because while we make the partial amend verbally, we silently make a full amend, a commitment to a changed behavior.

Steps Eight and Nine: Written Exercise

1. Explain how making amends will help you release the past. Why is this important?

2. What are your major fears about making amends? How can you overcome them?

3. What is the difference between an amend and an apology?

4. List three people to whom you need to make amends and explain why.

5. Write out your amend to yourself.

6. After yourself, what is the most important amend you can make?

7. Who will it be the most difficult to make amends to? Why?

8. Are there people to whom you feel you cannot make full amends? Who? Why can't you?

9. How can your Higher Power help you make amends?

Steps Eight and Nine: Imagery Exercise

Imagine you are making a list of people to whom you need to make amends. Ask your Higher Power for help. The list doesn't have to be absolutely complete; you can repeat this exercise as often as necessary.

Now choose someone on the list and carefully plan your amend with help from your Higher Power.

Now imagine being with the person to whom you will make the amend. Imagine the scene in as much detail as possible.

Now make your amend. If you feel afraid or have difficulty, ask your Higher Power for support. When you are finished, thank the person you harmed for hearing your amend and your Higher Power for staying with you.

Now take time to experience the feeling of having completed the amend. Then return to your day, knowing that this exercise will help you when the time comes to make the amend for real.

CHAPTER TWELVE

SPIRITUAL AWAKENING

Step Ten: Continued to take personal inventory and when we were wrong promptly admitted it.

In working Steps One through Nine we have learned to change our way of being. We have built a new spiritual base; we have both identified and identified with our pain. We have learned how to relieve the negative feelings that have controlled us and come to terms with our past. Our lives are now different, better. We have given up our attempts to control the outcome—we have learned to take responsibility only for the process and to trust that the process will take us where we need to go. We have a new will for loving. Most of us experience a new sense of peace, of comfort, of being in place. We are on the other side of Step Nine, and the question is how do we prevent relapse and continue our growth?

Jane explains how she feels: "Things are so different, I am so different. Sometimes I get scared I'll lose it."

Rhoda says: "I'm used to living by the program now. It's habit. I'm afraid that I'm not paying attention to it the way I should. I sure don't want to fall back to the way I was before."

Steps Ten through Twelve show us how to deal with what Jane and Rhoda are afraid of. In Step Ten, we can learn a method to maintain our new life pattern. Step Eleven can help us deepen our understanding and commitment. And Step Twelve can show us how to continue our growth by reaching beyond our own lives. These last three Steps ask for our commitment to continue work and that means a commitment to our growing spiritual strength and wellness. As we accept the program as a lifelong process, the need to immediately reach our goal diminishes and we relax into our new self.

Continued to take personal inventory . . .

Behavioral psychologists tell us that it takes at least six months to begin to integrate new thinking patterns or behavior into our lives. Even after that, we have urges to relapse. A recovering smoker will have an urge for a cigarette four, or even twenty-four years after he or she has stopped smoking. Stress, difficult times, or life crises can bring about old behavior. It seems that when things get tough, our oldest, most ingrained, and most familiar, gut-level feelings resurface and take over. Most of us understand this and watch out. But we also should be vigilant at ordinary times, when perhaps we have the flu or a cold, or we're tired, or haven't been eating well, when we're just not quite on. At these times, too, we're very vulnerable to fall back into our "favorite" emotional pain.

We need to keep the program at the front of our consciousness so we can *act* on it rather than *react* to negative circumstances. We need to develop small daily rituals that keep us constantly aware of our new pattern of living. Then we won't slip, by omission, back into our old painful, self-destructive ways.

Staying on Top

A.A. literature offers three techniques for maintaining consciousness of the program.

Spot Check Inventory: Several times a day we can stop and quickly review our feelings and behavior to see whether we have been following our new ways. In this way, we can make prompt repairs. Perhaps we need to refer back to the Third Step, or the

Fourth, or make an immediate amend. We do whatever seems appropriate, and we do it promptly. We can also use a spot check when a question or dilemma arises for which we don't have an easy answer. Then we take time to go back over what we have learned and respond accordingly. The more we can do this, the less we will find ourselves "losing it" to our old thoughts and actions.

Daily Inventory: The daily inventory serves a different purpose. This is a once-a-day review. It doesn't have to be long, or complicated, or time-consuming. We can do it as we are brushing our teeth, getting ready for bed, or perhaps just before we go to sleep. Doing this inventory ritually can remind us that the Twelve Steps is a program we live one day at a time. It keeps us focused on the present, today, and helps us give up anxiety about either the past or the future. We ask ourselves: *Did I feel an old familiar pain today? If so, what did I do about it? Could I have handled it differently, better? Do I need to make amends? If I do, when and how will I do it? Did I slip back into controlling, managing, or manipulating others? Did I truly surrender the outcome?* If we didn't, we need to do some Third Step work. The daily practice of this inventory helps us to maintain honesty and humility, and leads to continuing spiritual growth.

Long-Term Inventory: This inventory is done a few times a year. We set aside enough time for a comprehensive look at how we have been doing. We look at our progress from a long-term perspective, getting a clear picture of our gains and where we need to focus our work in the future. Many of us may like to use this time to celebrate our progress—and be thankful.

. . . and when we were wrong promptly admitted it.

We are going to relapse—some of us more than others. As we work the Twelve Steps we must accept that relapse is a part of our new life. Like a former smoker who has a few cigarettes, we can relapse into pain and the behavior that goes with it. It's inevitable. The Tenth Step is designed to help us realize that relapse is not the end of the world and helps us cope with that fact.

When we do a spot check and a daily inventory, we can catch relapses quickly and promptly repair them. Promptness is crucial. If we allow ourselves to drop back into our old ways, we are apt to feel guilty or ashamed over our relapse. But when we are prompt in making our repairs, feelings of guilt and shame can't drive us into a pit of self-hatred where we have to use denial, rationalization, and grandiosity to cover our disgust. These spirit destroyers don't have a chance to get rooted, so they can't undercut our spiritual healing. Remember, when we fall back to our old ways we haven't lost all that we gained. We just have to get back to doing the things that keep us emotionally healthy.

The Tenth Step is program maintenance. Here we recognize that we can relapse into emotional pain; we admit that we have a problem with old feelings and behaviors, and promptly make repairs. It is a point from which we can go back and recommit to what we already know and move forward to deepening and expanding our spirits.

Step Ten: Written Exercise

1. In doing the spot check and daily inventory, what emotional pains seem to keep reappearing?

2. Which of your old emotional pains seem to have disappeared?

3. What is the value of spot-check inventories?

4. What is the value of daily inventories?

5. What is the value of long-term inventories?

6. What does "The Tenth Step is the maintenance Step" mean to you?

7. Why does the Tenth Step help us toward spiritual growth one day at a time?

Step Ten: Imagery Exercise

Imagine yourself driving, taking a walk, washing dishes, exercising, taking a bath or shower, any ordinary activity—something you do every day, alone. Just be there with yourself.

Now do a spot-check inventory. Look back at your day so far and see how you are doing with emotional pain.

Now imagine that you remember feeling an old, familiar pain or behaving in a way that reflects a negative emotion. Decide what you need to do to repair the situation and release yourself from it. Take your time; do a complete job of repair.

Now reenter your day, keeping in mind the importance of the Tenth Step message.

CHAPTER THIRTEEN

GAINING PEACE

Step Eleven: Sought through prayer and meditation to improve our conscious contact with the God of our understanding, praying only for knowledge of God's will for us and the power to carry that out.

The purpose of the Eleventh Step is to reaffirm for us, each day, the first three Steps of the program. To admit our powerlessness, to recognize a healing Power outside of ourselves, and to turn our wills and our lives over to the care of that Power has given us the strength to turn our lives around. Now we have to keep it that way. This Step is our chance to develop an ever deepening awareness of our Higher Power and the peace that comes with that relationship. It is a daily recommitment to our spirituality.

Step Eleven works in tandem with the Tenth. As we carry out our spot check and daily inventories, we use conscious contact with our Higher Power to help and sustain us. And, like the inventories of Step Ten, daily meditation and prayer keeps the program in our consciousness and keeps it growing. We may feel a letdown when we have passed through the initial excitement and dedication to our new way of life—the Eleventh Step helps us deal with that. It's like love. First there is the romantic attraction, thrilling in its newness and possibility. Then this passes, and we are ready to begin to learn to deeply love, to become completely involved and intimate with our loved one, in good times and in bad. Living within the belief system of the Twelve Steps is the process of love, love for the very deepest and most important part of ourselves: our spiritual core.

Sought through prayer and meditation to improve our conscious contact with the God of our understanding, . . .

Three previous Steps have called for us to make "conscious contact" with our Higher Power. Step Three asked us to turn over our wills and our lives. Step Five asked us to admit our emotional pains, and Step Seven asked to have our pain removed. All these Steps involved direct, conscious communications with a Power greater than ourselves. Now Step Eleven seeks to improve that communication.

The method we choose to improve our "conscious contact" will differ, depending on our beliefs. Some of us will pray, some will meditate. It absolutely does not matter which form we use. As long as we are faithful in practicing whichever technique is comfortable for us and are humble and sincere, our relationship with our Higher Power can become stronger and we can increasingly find help.

In the Western world, the traditional way to contact our Higher Power is through prayer. Praying involves such things as asking for what we want and asking for guidance. Most of us start out learning prayers that ask for something important to us: "God bless Mommy and Daddy and Puff and Spot. Let Santa Claus bring me a new doll. Please don't let Grandma die." It's only later, as we move from the self-centeredness of childhood to more mature adults, that we can learn to say, "Thy will be done." Now as we work this Step we must keep in mind that, always, our request for guidance must supercede "I want . . ."—no matter how important the "I want" is.

Meg, who is blind says, 'I have a special time set aside every morning after I wake up but I'm still in bed and no one knows I'm awake when I spend a few minutes praying. I say 'The Serenity Prayer' and the 'Our Father.' Sometimes I pray for guidance about something in my life that I am dealing with; then I'm quiet and wait to see what I hear. I pray at other times during the day, too, and sometimes I just have conversations with God about something or other—but I never miss those morning prayers."

Those of us who were not raised in, or have moved away from, traditional religion, often use a different channel through which to communicate with our Higher Power. We may follow the Eastern practice of meditation. Meditation can help us learn to quiet our mind and rid us of the daily "noise" that fills our consciousness. When we remove the barriers of conscious thought, our Higher Power can enter our minds and in the stillness we can receive the guidance we ask for.

Jane tells us how she practices meditation: "I sit quietly and empty my mind of whatever confusion is there. I concentrate on relaxing my body too. Then I take a few deep breaths and let my White Light fill my mind. I just sit and look at it—and I always have healing thoughts come to me."

Dan's Higher Power is the program itself. This is how he explains his meditation. "I don't even like to call it meditating, but my friends tell me that's what I'm doing when I sit with my Higher Power. What I do is to be quiet, someplace by myself, and just think about the program, what it says and what it means to me. Nothing else, no particular problem, just the program. The thing that happens is that I always seem to have a part of it come to mind that turns out to be helpful in something that I'm dealing with in my life at that point. I've come to rely on it."

. . . praying only for knowledge of God's will for us and the power to carry that out.

Seeking guidance toward spiritual wellness is hard and may continue to cause us problems. It's so easy to fall back into rigidly trying to manage our lives and asking our Higher Power to support us in *our* will. Again and again we need to give up our attempts to control, accept our powerlessness, and seek guidance — it's our only way to the spiritual health we're looking for. Controlling keeps us focused outward, watching ourselves managing others. Step Eleven helps us increase our inward focus, and that focus becomes clearer through our Higher Power. It encourages our spirits to take root in the fertile soil of that internal relationship and become strong.

Spiritual growth can result from the awareness that our Higher Power's guidance should direct our lives, not our own willfulness. We can remember that our basic tasks are to be open-minded about reality and to be willing to change.

Anita, who lives with severe chronic asthma says, "I've struggled and struggled with this 'will' business. And I've come to think that maybe accepting my Higher Power's 'will for me' just means that I should accept reality as it is, without denial and without trying to control everything."

One side of Joe's face droops as a result of the stroke he suffered five years ago, but the other side lifts in a smile. He says, "I think the evidence that my prayers for guidance are answered shows up when I have opportunities to act in the old way and instead choose the new one. I figure that when I've done this enough times, the new way will become the old way, the old way will be gone, and I will have received guidance."

Anita and Joe describe the practical essence of the Eleventh Step. We can find the guidance of our Higher Power as we accept reality, without denial, and apply the Twelve Step program. In this way we can learn to cope with the stress of day-to-day living without emotional stress taking a toll. True acceptance of our reality can give us a sense of peace, even when that reality contains lots of difficult and active living. It's like Yoga exercises. We stretch and work our body while breathing deeply and focusing our minds on our quiet spiritual core. Although life may be very strenuous on the outside, it's very serene within.

Step Eleven: Written Exercise

1. What does prayer mean to you?

2. What does meditation mean to you?

3. Which (prayer or meditation) is the more comfortable method for you to use in your "conscious contact" with your Higher Power? Explain why.

4. What emotional roadblocks interfere with your deepening contact with your Higher Power? What do you need to do to get past them?

5. List three situations in which prayer or meditation has resulted in the guidance you asked for.

6. How do you see your Higher Power's will or guidance as present in your life today?

Step Eleven: Imagery Exercise

Imagine yourself sitting alone in a quiet, safe place. Relax and become comfortable. See yourself as ready to make "conscious contact" with your Higher Power.

Now imagine yourself carrying out the Eleventh Step, praying or meditating with your Higher Power. Experience the feeling. Take your time with this; imagine your complete prayer or meditation.

Now when you have finished your prayer or meditation, thank your Higher Power for giving you guidance.

Now come back to your day, remembering that whenever you need guidance about a concern, or simply feel the desire for contact, your Higher Power is always available to you.

SHARING OUR NEWFOUND PEACE

Step Twelve: Having had a spiritual awakening as the result of these steps, we tried to carry this message to others with chronic illness or disability, and to practice these principles in all our affairs.

When we started the Twelve Steps our goal was spiritual health despite our physical conditions. Now we have been introduced to the entire program—one Step at a time. We have carried out each Step to the best of our ability and are willing to commit ourselves to reworking them whenever necessary for the rest of our lives. And our lives may have changed. Today our real selves may be the selves we show the world; we no longer hide them under layers of emotional pain. Our behavior may have changed too. We may have better friendships and family life as we relate to others with honesty and humility. Our spirits are now rooted, growing strong and healthy. We know what it is to have moments of peace, serenity, and joy.

Having had a spiritual awakening as the result of these steps, . . .

Most of us are not exactly sure of how our spiritual awakening has come about. It may have started somewhere back in the first Steps and sort of happened along the way. We know that it can continue until we die. It's come out of an accumulation of mini-miracles and spiritual experiences that have resulted in joyful acceptance of our powerlessness and in faith that our Higher Power will truly care for us—always.

Meg has found a way to live with her Christian God and find peace. Jane has found a "path with heart," a Tao, which is a way to live in harmony with the universe.

Our spiritual awakenings have taken different forms, but we have found similar gifts. We have a new basis for living, knowing we aren't alone. We no longer need to be afraid of reality, neither the reality of who we are nor what our lives are like. And we can have confidence in our strength to continue this new way of being.

Our spiritual awakening may have been accompanied by a change in values. Perhaps we used to value isolation because it separated us from others and we could hide our pain. Now we value intimacy and connection with the world around us. Perhaps we used to value our denial because it supported our false reality. Now we value clarity and openness, in our relationships with others and with ourselves. Perhaps we used to value our anger as self-protection. Now we use its power as helpful energy for positive growth. Perhaps we used to value our powerlessness as a tool to manipulate others. Now we value it because it connects us to our Higher Power and leads to serenity.

. . . *we tried to carry this message to others with chronic illness or disability,* . . .

We now know how the program works. We have had our baptism of fire as we experienced it for ourselves, and now we need to carry its message beyond our own lives. Reaching out to others continues our growth, giving us increasing knowledge, new insights, intimacy, and the miracle of seeing other people change. And it's not hard to do. We don't need any special expertise, only humility and compassion. We pass on what we have learned by presenting ourselves and telling of our struggle— this can help others recognize their pain and need. Our story may give them a model for behavior and the gift of hope. And as we share with others, we may receive a gift too. We can see our old ways in people just beginning the program, and we can see how far we have come. We can watch others who have gone before us, and see how much more we can hope to accomplish.

One of the most effective ways to carry our message is to participate in groups of other chronically ill or disabled people.* Groups provide support, understanding, and empathy from those whose life experiences are much like our own—and who share the emotional pains we know so well. Groups are a place to learn to trust others to accept us as we are, even when we let it all out. As we allow others to know us, we are practicing and reaping the rewards of honesty. We get reality checks when we talk about our lives and people respond, reinforcing the beliefs of the

---

*See Appendix Four, "Finding a Mutual Aid Group."

Twelve Steps and helping us see where our denial may be misleading us. In groups we learn to accept our place without grandiosity. We are just a single person, in some ways so different, yet in basic ways no different, from all of the others. It's a true lesson in humility. We may be models for other group members, while at the same time we see them as models for our own use.

Groups can provide hope. We come to know others who grow and change; we see them become spiritually healthy, and we hear what difficult times they have had. Then we begin to see that our own circumstances, no matter how hard, can be dealt with, perhaps even turned into spiritually enriching experiences. And groups can be a wonderful support for the Eleventh Step. When we join together, we can make a kind of collective "conscious contact" with our individual Higher Powers. We consciously contact others with chronic illness or disabilities as we search for spiritual growth, and then we reinforce each individual's "conscious contact" with his or her Higher Power.

In *Living with a Chronic Illness,** Daniel Anderson presents seven suggestions for a successful self-help group.

1. Join with others who share your situation (in our case, others with chronic illness or disability).
2. Admit and accept your condition.
3. Surrender and admit that you, by yourself, are helpless to change the situation or condition that is limiting your life.
4. Since you are helpless, ask for help from some Higher Power and acknowledge your dependence on it.
5. Follow the group's basic Steps or suggested way of life. Get an experienced group member to guide you in the ways of the group.
6. Continually acknowledge that human beings are limited, that mutual interdependence is needed.

---

*Daniel Anderson. *Living with a Chronic Illness.* Center City, Minn.: Hazelden Educational Materials, 1986.

7. Keep in mind that "You alone can do it, but you can't do it alone."

. . . and to practice these principles in all our affairs.

This last requirement of Step Twelve asks that we live all we have learned. It asks that we keep each Step in our consciousness and faithfully practice the Tenth and Eleventh Steps every day of our lives. It suggests that when we have a problem or a concern we review program principles, applying them to our current situation, and shape our response in terms of what we find. What we have learned we must practice and then we will become. There is a story that may help us understand.

Once a well-known psychiatrist visited a Hopi Indian reservation. Something about the Indian mind fascinated him, and he thought that perhaps studying it would help his work. One day he was watching an old man weaving. The old man asked the psychiatrist what he did in the place he came from. The psychiatrist tried to explain that he worked with people's minds. The Hopi asked what that meant and the psychiatrist said that it was pretty complicated to explain but it had to do with people whose feelings and emotions didn't function right. The old man asked if the psychiatrist could heal these people. The psychiatrist said that depended on the diagnosis. The Hopi then commented that all healing was in the dance, the dance of life. Excited and intrigued by the idea, the psychiatrist asked if the old man would teach him the dance of life. And the Hopi said, "Yes, of course, I will teach you the steps, but you must bring your own music."

If we chronically ill and disabled people bring along the music of the Twelve Step program, we can be healed as we go through the dance of life.

Step Twelve: Written Exercise

1. How can a spiritual awakening affect your life?

2. Describe how the spiritual changes you've already experienced have affected the way you think and feel.

3. What is one way you plan to carry the message of the Twelve Steps to others with chronic illness or disability? How can this help them? How can this help you?

4. What could you gain from belonging to a group of others with chronic illness or disability?

Step Twelve: Imagery Exercise

Imagine yourself sitting comfortably in a group with several other people who are chronically ill or disabled. You are relaxed, pleased to be there.

Now imagine that you have decided to tell the group about your condition, about all of the emotional pain you have felt. As you talk, describe not only the pain but some of the things you did as a result.

Now explain how the Twelve Steps have helped you, how your life has changed. Also describe what parts of the Twelve Steps have seemed easy and what parts you have struggled with.

Now talk a little about what you see as your challenge to spiritual growth in the future.

When you have finished, ask if any of the others would like to respond to your story. If they do, listen to what they say. Don't argue, just hear them. Then thank them for giving you feedback and for listening to your story.

Now imagine yourself in a circle with the others, holding hands and repeating The Serenity Prayer.

> God grant me the serenity
> To accept the things I cannot change,
> The courage to change the things I can,
> And the wisdom to know the difference.

Now return to your day, knowing that, whenever you choose to, you can bring this image to life.

CHAPTER FOURTEEN

WHAT WILL HAPPEN

As we live the Twelve Steps, what happens can be awesome. Our illness or disability can become a beginning, a take-off point in our lives, rather than a dead end. We can find the beginning of a new self, a new life, a new sense of time. In the past we may have been imprisoned by our view of ourselves as ill or disabled "for the rest of our lives." Now we are freed from this constraint. Now we know that the rest of our lives can be lived one Step, one day, at a time. It is the fulfillment of the moment that matters, not what will someday be.

All humans go through life on a tightrope. Some of us are forced by circumstance to look down, and we are never the same as those who don't. We know, deep in our soul, the potential for vulnerability and catastrophe. For us, that potential has become real. Our chronic illness or disability has come to us and we know that it won't disappear. But we have found another way. We have found a way to live so that our spiritual growth becomes more important to us than our concern with chronic physical problems and emotional pain.

Many philosophers tell us that the growth of the spirit is the ultimate goal of human existence. It isn't the evolution of our bodies, or the extent of our accomplishment or material success that matters, but the growth of our souls—our spirituality. We chronically ill or disabled people are put in a position where we may have to look beyond our physical being for fulfillment, because our physical being is limited. But there are no limitations on the growth of our soul, and the Twelve Steps can guide us toward spiritual wellness. The beauty of this program is that it can work for anyone. It provides a way to accept the truth of a Higher Power without binding it in dogma. It loosens the boundaries of what is spiritual and therefore can embrace people of all religious and philosophical beliefs.

There are some specific goals we strive for on our journey toward spiritual fulfillment. We strive to receive strength and understanding from our Higher Power. We strive to surrender our self-centeredness and to practice honesty, humility, appreciation, and forgiveness. We strive to give service to others. And finally, we strive for balance.

We try for balance between our involvement with the process we live and surrendering the outcome of that process. We try to balance a focus on our Higher Power with our soul-searching. We are constantly trying to distinguish between "willfully taking control" of our lives and "being appropriately responsible for" them, as outlined by the Twelve Steps.

Too often we try to force the balance in our lives, rather than allowing ourselves room just to be balanced. We need to stay calm, to take it slowly, to quiet ourselves. Then we can find our center of balance, which leads us to peace, serenity, and joy. As ballet dancers or Yoga masters need balance in their spirits to move their bodies in unbelievable ways, so our spirits need balance to be fulfilled.

Accept the Twelve Step program as a way of life and we'll live happily ever after. Right? If only it were that simple. Yes, if we accept the Steps as our basis for living, we must work them for the rest of our lives. On one hand it gets even harder because we become so much more aware of ourselves, of the world around us, and of what our responses need to be. On the other, it gets easier as our new ways become more habitual and as we become more deeply aware of the support our Higher Power gives us.

The Serenity Prayer (which we can call The Serenity Meditation if we prefer) can help us as we grow. First, it teaches us that some things in our lives are beyond our control and some are even beyond our influence. Acceptance of the things we cannot change can lead us to serenity and open the door to a celebration of life.

Second, we receive the courage, dedication, and strength to take the responsibility for influencing those things that are not beyond our control—to change what we can. Both behavioral and spiritual change takes much strength and much courage. We have learned that while we cannot change our physical condition, we can change our attitude toward our bodies and the way we live our lives. We have looked at our emotional pain and found that a new spiritual approach can help us turn the negatives of anger, jealousy, and fear into positive, creative energy. In the past we may have anticipated change with fear and dread which blocked our going forward. Now we are learning that change offers the opportunity to focus on our spirituality and gives us a chance to grow.

Finally, we are beginning to understand the difference between what we can change and what we cannot. Listening closely to the voice of our Higher Power helps us differentiate between the two. With our Higher Power's help, we can use all we know to stay with reality, to fight off the denial and rationalization that supports our past ways.

In addition to The Serenity Prayer, there are other thoughts we use. We strive to:

Surrender the outcome. Picture a spider web: small, delicate, yet strong, spun across the corner of a kitchen baseboard. It's hardly noticeable, but a drama is taking place there that is important for us to watch. A small, unsuspecting fly flits near the web, veers too close, and gets caught. As the fly struggles, the spider, which has left the web to crawl across the kitchen floor, begins to scurry back to eat its victim. But a Siamese cat, blue eyes flashing, sable tail twitching, stalks the spider. As the cat is about to pounce on his tasty snack, a woman steps into the corner, crushing the spider and tearing down the web. The cat sits back on his haunches, staring at the woman. A small drama, almost meaningless. Or is it? What can this tiny incident teach us about control, about outcomes?

The fly had no way of knowing that it would be caught in a web. The spider had no way of knowing that it was being stalked by a cat. The cat had no way of knowing that his mistress would destroy his treat. And this is true for all of us, all of the time. We have no way of knowing. But we worry, and we fret, and we try to control our outcomes, using precious energy, perhaps working in direct contradiction to the Twelve Steps. The fly, the spider, and the cat certainly didn't seem concerned about the outcomes in their lives, and it wouldn't have mattered if they had been. They had no control, and ultimately, neither do we. We need to surrender the outcome, to stop worrying, and to use our energy to be the very best we can for the moment that we have.

We can do our utmost to concentrate on each moment and whatever task or event is at hand. We can approach the moments of our life with love and openness to their potential. We can live in the present, not in the past or the future. We can do this when we trust where the process is taking us, believing that wherever our lives go we will have the opportunity for spiritual growth. We can, with serenity, surrender the outcome. As a result, we drop our anxiety about the past and the future and concentrate on our moment in life. And that's really all there is—the rest is nonreality. What has been, was; what will be, is not yet.

Have the will for loving. We've learned that love isn't just romance or eros (the desire for sensual relationships). We've learned that loving is extending ourselves to nurture our own or another's spiritual growth. This means that life can be full of love, for ourselves, for our intimate friends and family, and for many other people whose paths we cross. We love ourselves when we are soft with ourselves, when we take time out to rest and reflect, when we treat ourselves to a new dress or pants, a trip, a special time with a friend. We find self-love when we pray, or meditate, or walk in a dew-covered garden in the morning. And we love ourselves when we are tough with ourselves too— when we don't let ourselves get caught in our old pain, but force ourselves to attend to the new things we know, even though it would be so much easier to lapse back. We love ourselves when we focus our anger realistically, when we push ourselves to confront a fearful situation, and when we stand up for ourselves with our doctor, or boss, or loved one.

We can love others by hugging them and telling them they're terrific. We also love them when we confront them with their self-destructive behavior or about a problem in the relationship between us. At these times, we love them even when what we do makes them angry or they reject us. Our love shows in the process, not the outcome.

Love takes willpower, patience, attention, concentration, kindness, thoughtfulness, understanding, empathy, and toughness. Loving is hard; it takes so much energy, so much time. But loving is easier when we know that we are loved, that there is a Power greater than ourselves that unfailingly cares for us. As this sense of love grows in our lives, we can share it with others. We have a model of being loved which we, in turn, can use to nurture those around us.

Stay open to the possibilities in each moment of our day. Until now, most of us have never done this. Even though we understand the words, it may be a hard idea to comprehend. Each moment of each day contains a myriad of possibilities. Each moment connects the past and the future. It brings the experience and knowledge acquired in the past into the present so we can make choices that will influence our future. What life really comes down to is choice. No matter what happens to us, as long as we are in a physically conscious state we retain the power of choice. We can choose to recognize a Power greater than ourselves or we can choose to go it alone.

We can choose to accept grace or to ignore its existence. We can choose to struggle toward perfection or to accept our human limitations. We have a choice of what to perceive, what decisions to make, what thoughts to think about what is happening, what feelings to have, and each choice will lead to a different outcome.

Take this moment as an example. You can choose to continue to read this book and to accept what it's saying about the importance and potential of each moment. You can feel excited about the prospect of enlarging your awareness in this way. This attitude may lead to behaviors that can broaden your life and experience. Or you can choose to be skeptical, saying, "Well, I don't know about this, but I'll think about it." Or you can choose to close the book, saying, "Bunch of junk." Each of these responses will lead to a different outcome. But whether we choose to close the book, question it, or believe its message, the reality is that this moment is all we have of life. We mentally recycle the past, holding on to its problems and its pain, we fantasize about the future, dreaming outcomes based on fear or desire, but we can only live the moment we are in.

An old saying goes, "We only live for an instant, so make the best of it." This is generally understood to mean that within the greater scheme of things our individual life is very short, so we better live as well as we can. But it can also mean that there is no past and no future, only the *instant,* that moment when life happens. This instant is the only time we have to think, to feel, to act, and to choose. The exciting part is that each moment is a crossroads, full of potential for growth, change, or stagnation. We need only to stay open to the possibilities that it presents. And when life is hard, when we don't know how we can stand to go on, it helps to know that each instant in which we live is very short, that we can certainly handle this one tiny space of time.

Be present for the acceptance of joy, of peace, and of grace or enlightenment. It's as if we are a jigsaw puzzle. We began the Twelve Steps with pieces of ourselves lying around, mixed up, some even upside down. We arranged the pieces; slowly, beginning with the edges, we filled ourselves in, and our picture took shape. Finally we are left with only one piece to drop in, just one, in the very center of our puzzle. We pick it up and fit it in. This is the piece that lives at our core. Grace is the Christian word for it; others call it Enlightenment; still others, Joy or Peace. But the name doesn't matter. It is the powerful force that originates outside of human consciousness and that supports and protects and enhances the spiritual growth of human beings. This central piece contains the light that we carry within us. We can never control how dark it may get on the outside, but with this final part of ourselves in place, our inner light will always show us the way.

APPENDIX ONE

THE TWELVE STEPS FOR
CHRONICALLY ILL OR DISABLED PEOPLE*

1. We admitted we were powerless over chronic illness—our lives had become unmanageable.
2. Came to believe that a Power greater than ourselves could restore us to sanity.
3. Made a decision to turn our will and our lives over to the care of God *as we understood Him*.
4. Made a searching and fearless moral inventory of ourselves.
5. Admitted to the God of our understanding, to ourselves, and to another human being the exact nature of our wrongs.
6. Were entirely ready to have the God of our understanding remove all of our defects of character.
7. Humbly asked God to remove our shortcomings.
8. Made a list of all persons we had harmed, and became willing to make amends to them all.
9. Made direct amends to such people wherever possible, except when to do so would injure them or others.
10. Continued to take personal inventory and when we were wrong promptly admitted it.
11. Sought through prayer and meditation to improve our conscious contact with the God of our understanding, praying only for knowledge of God's will for us and the power to carry that out.
12. Having had a spiritual awakening as the result of these steps, we tried to carry this message to others with chronic illness or disability, and to practice these principles in all our affairs.

---

*Adapted from the Twelve Steps of Alcoholics Anonymous, reprinted with permission of A.A. World Services, Inc., New York, N.Y.

APPENDIX TWO

THE TWELVE STEPS OF ALCOHOLICS ANONYMOUS*

1. We admitted we were powerless over alcohol—that our lives had become unmanageable.
2. Came to believe that a Power greater than ourselves could restore us to sanity.
3. Made a decision to turn our will and our lives over to the care of God *as we understood Him.*
4. Made a searching and fearless moral inventory of ourselves.
5. Admitted to God, to ourselves, and to another human being the exact nature of our wrongs.
6. Were entirely ready to have God remove all these defects of character.
7. Humbly asked Him to remove our shortcomings.
8. Made a list of all persons we had harmed, and became willing to make amends to them all.
9. Made direct amends to such people wherever possible, except when to do so would injure them or others.
10. Continued to take personal inventory and when we were wrong promptly admitted it.
11. Sought through prayer and meditation to improve our conscious contact with God *as we understood Him,* praying only for knowledge of His will for us and the power to carry that out.
12. Having had a spiritual awakening as the result of these steps, we tried to carry this message to alcoholics, and to practice these principles in all our affairs.

---

*The Twelve Steps are taken from *Alcoholics Anonymous* (Third Edition), published by A.A. World Services, Inc., New York, N.Y., pp. 59-60. Reprinted with permission.

APPENDIX THREE

DAILY MEDITATIONS*

TODAY:

I will take a good look at myself and realize that I have many emotional pains that have become dominant in my life. I am at the mercy of my pain and unable to manage it. Understanding this, I admit that I need help.

I will acknowledge the presence of a Power greater than myself that is fully capable of healing my pain.

I will let go of my need to be physically "normal," and will focus instead on my spiritual growth. I will realize that my spiritual wellness can supercede my physical problems, that spiritual growth is the ultimate goal of humankind.

I will let go of my inclination to analyze and question my situation. I will surrender myself to live by the tenets of the Twelve Step recovery program. While I will continue to make my own life happen, I will accept that it is a Power greater than myself that shows me the way.

I will release the past, forgiving myself and others for the ways we have been. Searching for fault, or blaming myself and others, keeps me stuck in the past.

I will drop my anxiety about the future. I will live this day with as much joy, trust, and serenity as I can, realizing that this day is all that I can handle.

---

*Adapted with permission from *12 Steps for Adult Children.* San Diego: Recovery Publications, 1987.

I will concentrate on staying present in each moment, knowing that it is the only time I really have, the only time that I can effect change and growth in my life, the only time I can *act* toward my spiritual wellness.

I will take responsibility for all aspects of my life: my choices, my behavior, my feelings, my physical and mental health, my spiritual well-being, and the principles and values by which I live.

I will consciously use all my energies that contribute to the betterment of my life and the lives of others, such as expressing kindness, honesty, and integrity.

I will replace my negative thoughts with positive thoughts, knowing that this leads to my spiritual growth.

I will be grateful for the opportunity to be set free from old attitudes and behaviors that prevent me from moving toward spiritual healing.

I will fully accept myself, just as I am, loving myself and realizing my value and worthiness to others.

I will willingly share with others the wisdom, peace, and strength I have received through the Twelve Step program.

I will go forth into this day with enthusiasm and with the determination to enjoy it and give it my positive best, come what may.

FINDING A MUTUAL AID GROUP

The groups that we generally call self-help groups are probably better called groups for mutual aid. Their underlying principle is that people help themselves by helping each other, and that the helper gets as much from the giving as the person who is helped.

Finding a mutual aid group is not difficult. Many states and provinces have their own clearinghouses where people can go to get information about groups in their specific locality.

The following list is printed with permission of the Self-Help Clearinghouse, St. Clares-Riverside Medical Center, Denville, New Jersey. It originally appeared on pages 17-19 of *The Self Help Sourcebook*, written and edited by E. Madard and A. Meese and published in 1986.

Self-Help Clearinghouses

(CA) CALIFORNIA SELF-HELP
CENTER
University of California Los Angeles
405 Hilgard Avenue
Los Angeles, CA 90024
(213) 825-1799 or 800-222-LINK
Provides information on local
clearinghouses in the state, other
than those listed below.

(CA) SACRAMENTO SELF-HELP
CLEARINGHOUSE
Mental Health Association
of Sacramento
5370 Elvos Avenue, Suite B
Sacramento, CA 95819
(916) 456-2070

(CA) SAN FRANCISCO SELF-HELP
CLEARINGHOUSE
Mental Health Association
2398 Pine Street
San Francisco, CA 94115
(415) 921-4401

(CA) SELF-HELP
CLEARINGHOUSE OF
MERCED COUNTY
Mental Health Association of
Merced County
P.O. Box 343
Merced, CA 95341
(209) 723-8861

(CT) CONNECTICUT SELF-HELP/
MUTUAL SUPPORT NETWORK
Consultation Center
19 Howe Street
New Haven, CT 06511
(203) 789-7645

(IL) ILLINOIS SELF-HELP CENTER
1600 Dodge Avenue
Suite S-122
Evanston, IL 60201
(312) 328-0470

(KS) KANSAS SELF-HELP
NETWORK
Campus Box 34
Wichita State University
Wichita, KS 67208-1595
(316) 689-3170

(MA) CLEARINGHOUSE OF
MUTUAL HELP GROUPS
Massachusetts Cooperative
Extension
113 Skinner Hall
University of Massachusetts
Amherst, MA 01003
(413) 545-2313

(MI) MICHIGAN SELF-HELP
CLEARINGHOUSE
Michigan Protection & Advocacy
Service
109 West Michigan Avenue
Suite 900
Lansing, MI 48933
(517) 484-7373 or
1-800-752-5858 (for MI only)

(MI) CENTER FOR SELF-HELP
Riverwood Center
1485 Highway M-139
Benton Harbor, MI 49022
(616) 925-0594

(MN) MINNESOTA MUTUAL HELP
RESOURCE CENTER
Wilder Foundation Community
Care Unit
919 LaFond Avenue
St. Paul, MN 55104
(612) 642-4060

(MO) KANSAS CITY SUPPORT
GROUP CLEARINGHOUSE
Kansas City Association for Mental
Health
1020 East 63rd Street
Kansas City, MO 64110
(816) 361-5007

(NE) NEBRASKA SELF-HELP
INFORMATION SERVICES
1601 Euclid Avenue
Lincoln, NE 68502
(402) 476-9668

(NJ) NEW JERSEY SELF-HELP
CLEARINGHOUSE
St. Clare's Riverside Medical Center
Pocono Road
Denville, NJ 07834
(201) 625-9565 or
800-367-6274 (in NJ only)

(NY) NEW YORK STATE SELF-
HELP CLEARINGHOUSE
N.Y. Council on Children and Families
Empire State Plaza, Tower Building
Albany, NY 12223
(518) 474-6293
Also provides information on
additional local self-help
clearinghouses in the state other
than those listed below.

(NY) LONG ISLAND SELF-HELP
CLEARINGHOUSE
New York Institute of Technology
Central Islip Campus
Central Islip, NY 11722
(516) 348-3030

(NY) NEW YORK CITY SELF-HELP
CLEARINGHOUSE, INC.
P.O. Box 022812
Brooklyn, NY 11202
(718) 596-6000

(NY) WESTCHESTER SELF-HELP
CLEARINGHOUSE
Westchester Community College
Academic Arts Building
75 Grasslands Road
Valhalla, NY 10595
(914) 347-3620

(NY) NATIONAL SELF-HELP
CLEARINGHOUSE
City University of New York
Graduate Center
Room 1206A
33 W. 42nd Street
New York, NY 10036
(212) 840-1259

(OR) NORTHWEST REGIONAL
SELF-HELP CLEARINGHOUSE
718 W. Burnside Avenue
Portland, OR 97209
(503) 222-5555

(PA) SELF-HELP GROUP
NETWORK OF THE PITTSBURGH
AREA
710½ South Avenue
Wilkensburg, PA 15221
(412) 247-5400

(PA) SELF-HELP INFORMATION &
NETWORKING EXCHANGE
S.H.I.N.E., Voluntary Action Center
of N.E. Penn.
225 N. Washington Avenue
Park Plaza, Lower Level
Scranton, PA 18503
(717) 961-1234

(SC) MIDLAND AREA SUPPORT
NETWORK
Lexington Medical Center
2720 Sunset Blvd.
West Columbia, SC 29169
(803) 791-9227

(TX) DALLAS SELF-HELP
CLEARINGHOUSE
Mental Health Association
of Dallas County
2500 Maple Avenue
Dallas, TX 75201-1998
(214) 871-2420

(VT) VERMONT SELF-HELP
CLEARINGHOUSE
c/o Parents Assistance Line
103 South Main Street
.Waterbury, VT 05676
(802) 241-2249 or (Vermont only)
800-442-5356

(VA) GREATER WASHINGTON, D.C.
SELF-HELP COALITION
Mental Health Association
of N. Virginia
100 N. Washington Street
Suite 232
Falls Church, VA 22046
(703) 536-4100

(CANADA) CALGARY-FAMILY LIFE
EDUCATION COUNCIL
12th Avenue S.W.
Calgary, Alberta, Canada T2R 0G9
(403) 262-1117

(CANADA) SASKATCHEWAN SELF-
HELP DEVELOPMENT UNIT
410 Cumberland Avenue North
Saskatoon, Saskatchewan, 57M 1M6
(306) 652-7817

(CANADA) TORONTO – SELF-HELP
CLEARINGHOUSE OF METRO
40 Orchard View Blvd., Suite 215
Toronto, Ontario, Canada M4R 1B9
(416) 487-4355

(CANADA) WINNEPEG – SELF-
HELP RESOURCE
CLEARINGHOUSE
NorWest Coop & Health Center
103-61 Tyndall Avenue
Winnepeg, Manitoba, Canada R2X
2T4
(204) 589-5500 or 633-5955

BIBLIOGRAPHY

Anderson, Daniel. *Living with a Chronic Illness.* Center City, Minn.: Hazelden Educational Materials, 1986.

Burnett, Frances. *Secret Garden.* New York: Lippincott, J.B. Junior Books, 1962.

E., Stephanie. *Shame Faced.* Center City, Minn.: Hazelden Educational Materials, 1986.

Friedman, Meyer and Ray H. Rosenman. *A Behavior and Your Heart.* Greenwich, Conn.: Fawcett Inc., 1974.

Gartner, Alan and Frank Riessman. *The Self-Help Revolution.* New York: Human Services Press, 1982.

Kübler-Ross, Elisabeth. *On Death and Dying.* New York: Macmillan Publishing Co., Inc., 1969.

Kushner, Harold S. *When Bad Things Happen To Good People.* New York: Schocken Books, 1981.

Lerner, Rokelle. *Affirmations.* Pompano Beach, Fla.: Health Communications, Inc., 1985.

Peck, M. Scott. *The Road Less Traveled.* New York: Simon and Schuster, 1978.

Promoting Health, Preventing Disease: Objectives for the Nation. Washington, D.C.: U.S. Dept. of Health and Human Services, 1980.

Rossi, Ernest Lawrence. *The Psychobiology of Mind-Body Healing.* New York: W. W. Norton & Co., Inc., 1986.

Selye, Hans. *Stress Without Distress.* New York: New American Library, Inc., 1974.

Siegel, Bernie. *Love, Medicine, and Miracles.* New York: Harper and Row, 1986.

The Little Red Book. Center City, Minn.: Hazelden Educational Materials, 1970.

Touchstones. Center City, Minn.: Hazelden Educational Materials, 1986.

Viorst, Judith. *Necessary Losses.* New York: Balantine Books, 1986.

INDEX

A

A.A. Meeting, 53
Acceptance, 27, 44
Affirmations, 106
Alcoholics Anonymous, recovery program,
    3, 29, 31-32, 105
Ambiguity, 22-24, 71-74
Amends, how to make, 111-120
Amputee, 69, 77
Anger, 21-22, 26, 69-71
Anxiety, 18-19, 64-66
Arthritis, debilitating, 66, 80
Asthma, severe chronic, 130
Athiest, 42
Authority figures, 73

B

Balance, in our lives, 138
Balance, psychological, 78
Barriers, how to overcome, 54-55
Barriers, mental, 40
Barriers, physical, 27
Behavior patterns, 108
Behaviors, destructive, 96
Behaviors, habitual, 107-108
Behaviors, new, 108
Beliefs, cultural, 28
Blame, 22-24, 71-74
Blindness, 51-52, 64, 100, 128
Boundaries, 14
Breast cancer, 33, 69, 72
Bypass surgery, 72

C

Care, 50
Catharsis, emotional, 78, 100
Cerebral palsy, 19, 34, 66
Challenge, 8-9, 11, 14
Change, 8, 14, 25, 77
Chemotherapy, 12
Choice, the power of, 141
Chronic grief, 26
Colitis, 107

Commitment, public, 97, 114
Control, 4, 17, 36, 84, 140

D

Defects of character, 102
Denial, 24, 26, 29, 34, 58, 83, 111, 130,
    139
Depression, 51
Differences, 6, 24
Dishonesty, 57, 83

E

Emotional storms, 78
Emotions, spirit-enhancing, 92
Energy, 22, 49, 87, 139, 141
Enlightenment, 142-143
Envy, 24
Exhaustion, 27-28, 80-82

F

Faith, 51, 90
Family life, 132
Fatigue, emotional, 80
Fault, 23
Fear, 7-8, 18-19, 64-66, 111
Feelings, negative, 28
Freedom, 46, 81
Friends, their response, 13, 84, 132

G

God, 42, 128
Grace, 142-143
Grandiosity, 124
Grief, 25-27, 77-80
Groundwork, 47

H

Habits, 14, 108
Handicaps, accepting them, 7-8
Healing, 135
Heart attacks, 69

Heart disease, 42, 53
Higher Power, 38-46, 50, 54-55, 109
Higher Power, communicating with, 110,
   128-129, 139
Hope, 87-88
Humility, 32, 38, 62, 70, 100, 106-107, 115

I

Illness, hidden, 12
Immune system, 2
Inner light, 143
Insanity, 43
Intimacy, 74
Intolerance, 83
Introspection, 103
Inventory, daily, 123-124
Inventory, long-term, 123-124
Inventory, spot check, 122-125
Involvement, with others, 20
Isolation, 19-21, 66-68, 100

J

Jealousy, 24-25, 74-76
Joy, 29, 89-90, 142-143

K

Kidney disease, 41

L

Leukemia, 88
Limits, transcending them, 15, 54
Loneliness, way out of, 100
Losses, grieving them, 113
Love, 88-89, 140-141

M

Managing, 36
Manipulation, 114
Mastectomies, 42
Meditation, 127, 129, 141
Meditations, daily, 149-150
Melanoma, 107
Miracles, 90

Moment, living in the, 142
Mortality, accepting it, 7
Multiple sclerosis, 34, 80
Mutual aid groups, 133-134

O

Obsession, 75
Obstacles, 14
Osteoporosis, 69-70
Others, effects on, 11-12

P

Pain, cycle of, 28
Pain, emotional, 16-17, 26, 31, 45, 59, 72-
   73, 109
Pain, finding and facing, 58-59
Pain, removing it, 105
Painkillers, 52-53
Panic, 72
Paralyzed, 74
Parkinson's disease, 7, 28
Peace, 121, 142-143
Perfection, 5-6, 31
Philosophy, personal, 47
Possibilities, staying open to, 141
Power, 12-13, 35
Power, tools of, 104
Powerlessness, 17-18, 33-37, 61-63, 80
Powerlessness, as a manipulation, 114
Prayer, 127-128, 141
Pride, false, 57, 84
Pride, sapping energy, 36
Prophecies, negative, 88

Q

Quadriplegic, 26, 71

R

Rage, 21-22, 69-71
Rationalization, 69
Reality, 5
Rejection, 6
Relapse, 123-124
Relationships, 12-13

Relaxation, 53
Relief, 39
Religions, 28, 52, 54
Resentment, 24
Restrictions, 13-14
Rheumatoid arthritis, 52, 98
Risk, 98
Rituals, daily, 122
Roadblocks, 45

S

Self-awareness, 58, 60
Self-centeredness, 53, 57
Self-involvement, excessive, 84
Self-pity, 83
Self-respect, 109
Self-sufficiency, 40
Serenity, 29, 64, 91
Serenity, The Prayer, 106, 136, 139
Shame, 66
Solitude, 67
Spiritual awakening, 131-132
Spiritual force, connecting with, 47
Spiritual growth, 3-4, 8-9, 14, 33, 44, 54, 64, 88-89, 105, 130, 137, 143
Spiritual health, 78-79, 105, 129
Spirituality, 8-9, 41-46
Step One, 33-39
Step Two, 39-46
Step Three, 47-55
Step Four, 57-85
Step Five, 95-102

Step Six, 102-106
Step Seven, 60, 106-110
Step Eight, 111-114
Step Nine, 115-120
Step Ten, 121-125
Step Eleven, 127-131
Step Twelve, 131-136
Stress, emotional, 1
Stress, physical, 91
Stroke, 27, 130
Support groups, 133-134
Surrender, 35-37, 134, 139-140

T

Turning it over, 48-49
Twelve Step message, 136
Twelve Step process, 41
Twelve Step program, 3-4, 29, 31-32, 59, 63, 105, 113, 138, 142-143

V

Visualizing, 23-24
Vulnerability, physical, 81

W

Weaknesses, 65
Wellness, 112
White Light, 48, 129
Wounds, 6-7